Tough Decisions

TOUGH DECISIONS

Cases in Medical Ethics

SECOND EDITION

JOHN M. FREEMAN, M.D.
The Johns Hopkins Medical Institutions

KEVIN MCDONNELL, Ph.D.
Saint Mary's College, Notre Dame

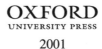

OXFORD
UNIVERSITY PRESS

2001

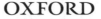

OXFORD

UNIVERSITY PRESS

Oxford   New York
Athens   Auckland   Bangkok   Bogotá   Buenos Aires   Calcutta
Cape Town   Chennai   Dar es Salaam   Delhi   Florence   Hong Kong   Istanbul
Karachi   Kuala Lumpur   Madrid   Melbourne   Mexico City   Mumbai
Nairobi   Paris   São Paulo   Shanghai   Singapore   Taipei   Tokyo   Toronto   Warsaw

and associated companies in
Berlin   Ibadan

Copyright © 2001 by John M. Freeman and Kevin McDonnell

Published by Oxford University Press, Inc.,
198 Madison Avenue, New York, New York, 10016
http://www.oup-usa.org

Library of Congress Cataloging-in-Publication Data
Freeman, John Mark.
Tough decisions : cases in medical ethics /
John M. Freeman, Kevin McDonnell.—2nd ed. p. ; cm.   Includes bibliographical references.
ISBN 0-19-509041-1 (cloth)—ISBN 0-19-509042-X (pbk.)
1. Medical ethics—Case studies.
2. Clinical medicine—Decision making—Case studies.
3. Decision making—Moral and ethical aspects—Case studies.
I. McDonnell, Kevin.
II. Title.
[DNLM: 1. Ethics, Medical.
2. Clinical Medicine.
3. Decision Making.
W 50 F855t 2001]   R725.5.F74 2001   174'.2—dc21   00-035945

2 4 6 8 9 7 5 3 1

Printed in the United States of America
on acid-free paper

We dedicate this book to the many children and their parents who, as we have struggled together through difficult times and tough decisions, have taught us to be better, wiser, and more humble decision makers.

We further dedicate this book to our wives, Elaine and Carol, and to our children for their forbearance while we have learned, taught, and written.

Preface

This book is about the difficult moral decisions that arise ever more frequently in the course of medical practice. The dilemmas we depict in this book are not the only moral issues in medicine, and possibly not even the most common, but they are among the most dramatic. Although we have presented them as fictional cases in order to explore their many nuances, they all originate from first-hand experience. They represent amalgams of true cases we have seen, discussed in depth, and sometimes personally managed. Some are like the dramatic cases played out in the newspapers or on nightly television, but in this book we do not allow the reader merely to look on while others decide: We cast the reader in the role of decision maker. What happens depends in part on the reader's decisions.

The book's format is intended to give readers a clear sense of the pressures that come to bear on clinical decision making. The cases are interrupted at critical points, and the reader is asked to make a decision. That choice at times leads to one of several paths through the case. Thus, as in real life, people have a role in shaping the course of events and sometimes the outcome. We assume that the reader wants to do the right thing but faces the problem of determining what that is. The dialogue of the cases embodies perspectives grounded in various moral theories, offering different views of what is right in given medical situations.

This book is not intended for ethicists, nor for philosophers or theologians. Each of us—parents, grown children, friends, and counselors—will, at some time, be faced with tough decisions. This book is intended for those of us faced with such decisions in the course of our actual lives.

In the second edition, we have organized the cases to follow the life cycle—running backward. We begin with issues surrounding death, since they are the most widely discussed topics in medical ethics today. We then proceed from adulthood to childhood to issues of conception and genetic planning. The organization of cases along this timeline is not rigid, however. For example, we discuss the allocation of scarce medical resources in the context of a case dealing with adolescent patients. The basic issues of medical ethics—good care for patients, informed consent, the fair allocation of social resources, etc.—occur at every stage of life.

This book is the fruit of a dialogue between a philosopher and a physician, a theorist and a clinician about the practice and teaching of medical ethics. The traditional teaching of ethics starts by laying a foundation in ethical theory and then applying one or more of the theories to carefully selected and articulated cases. Such an approach seems too academic and removed from reality. An alternative approach presents cases, each one illustrating a single moral theory or medical ethical situation. We found such case presentations to be cramped and artificial, similar to cases before an appellate court and lacking the drama, subtlety, and conflict of the original situation. They are often too brief to provide a sufficient sense of the interconnections between moral, medical, and social problems. There seemed to be no better solution than to write our own book.

There was a time when it was easier for physicians to decide what to do. They followed the Hippocratic oath, which says: "I will follow that regimen which, according to my ability and judgment, I consider for the benefit of my patients, and abstain from whatever is deleterious and mischievous." When the oath was written, few effective remedies were available. So long as they refrained from intentionally doing harm, physicians could be said to practice "good medicine." Advances in medical science and technology, however, have enabled physicians to prolong life or cure disease for many patients who were formerly beyond help. We now find ourselves asking whether there are situations in which the use of life-prolonging therapies may not be beneficial, or may even be harmful. We sometimes ask ourselves if the best course of action is to do nothing.

Nonetheless, it remains a basic tenet of medicine that physicians must always care for their patients. But the term "to care" is often misused in medical parlance as a synonym for "to treat," that is, to intervene or to do something active—starting a respirator, prescribing drugs or beginning tube feeding. There is an important distinction between the care and concern that should always be provided and these technical interventions.

Having stated the obvious—that physicians must always care for their patients and do what is to their benefit—how do we define "benefit?" Beyond the minimum care required to sustain the dignity of a human being, the meaning of the word depends on the facts of the individual case and the interpretation and understanding of those facts by physicians, patients, families, and society.

Two factors have heightened the problematic character of the decisions we now face in medicine. The first is the development and widespread availability of new technology. It is now possible to transplant hearts and kidneys, to maintain breathing and heartbeat with a respirator, to save one-pound babies, and to assess an individual's likely future through DNA testing. We may soon be able to engineer that future by manipulating the human genome. In just a few years such methods will move from speculative gleams in the eyes of a few researchers to well-established and widely available therapies. The future promises to be even more awesome.

As the ability to perform "medical miracles" improves, we more frequently face moral questions about the development of technology and its legitimate use. Should we put a virtually brain dead patient on a respirator? Should we try one more therapy for a patient's cancer? Should we operate on a newborn child with many severe problems? Do such procedures benefit the patient or do they merely prolong misery? Should parents be allowed to select certain characteristics for their offspring? These are not technical questions but human and moral ones of the highest order.

Hand in hand with advances in technology have come changes in social attitudes toward medicine and the practice of medicine. Very few people are fortunate enough to have family physicians who have known and cared for them over long periods of time, physicians whose attitudes and values they know and share. The great mobility of North Americans and the fact that more and more conditions are treated by specialists have made it less likely that health care providers will know the attitudes and the moral and values diversity of their patients and the effects of their diversity on medical decision making. In addition, many patients and their families want to be better informed and to participate more actively in their health care decisions.

Many difficult medical decisions arise, therefore, from the increasing ambiguity that technology has introduced, and their difficulty is multiplied by increasing public and private conflicts over which courses of action are morally appropriate. Equally good and reasonable people confronting the same dilemma may reach different conclusions and take different actions.

We start with the assumption that most of us are basically decent people. But often individuals are unwittingly insensitive to, or unaware of, the moral issues involved in their decisions. Ethical theories can guide us, but using these theories well requires some grounding in ethics, some awareness of the context of the arguments and theories of good decision making.

Moral philosophy—ethics—has worked to develop organized ways of approaching these questions using, among many, the theories of Aristotle, the great classical Greek philosopher; Immanuel Kant, the German thinker at the center of the Enlightenment; and Utilitarian philosophers of nineteenth century Britain. Ethicists—philosophers and theologians—are students and interpreters of these varied approaches, many working to develop moral guidance for modern problems.

PREFACE

Even without knowing or appealing explicitly to ethical theory, health care professionals justify their decisions in terms of rights, duties, benefits, or some other staple of moral philosophy. Even when appealing to our feelings and intuitions or invoking the Hippocratic oath and professional obligations, people are using philosophical concepts. There is no way to morally justify a decision without using some of the elements and language of ethical theory.

In justifying their actions, some physicians focus on what will happen, that is, the outcome. Others want to designate a particular person—the patient, the parent or family, or the courts—who will make the decision. In the concluding chapters of this book, we argue that *how* the decision is made is most important; it is the process of decision making that counts.

Health care professionals are sometimes frustrated because they ask too much of ethicists, desiring specific answers to immediate problems. And they ask not just the standard questions like, "Should I treat this newborn infant?" or "Should I turn off Mr. X's respirator?" but also more subtle questions like, "How can I present the information to parents so they make the appropriate decision?" and "What are my responsibilities when the family or relatives are making what I believe is the wrong decision?" Ethics is not designed to answer specific questions like these. Rather, ethical theory offers a framework for thinking through decisions. It attempts to delineate the boundaries of morally acceptable behavior and illuminate the guidelines for making decisions within those boundaries. We believe that ethical theory is meant to tell us how to make a decision and what the ingredients and bases of a morally acceptable decision are, not what decision to make.

A further reason for the health care professional's frequent impatience with ethics is the pressure of time on the physician's decision-making process. In many situations a decision must be made without full information. Inability to decide or a delay engendered by a prolonged search for missing elements may constitute a decision by default. During the delay the patient may die or the opportunity for intervention may pass.

To simulate situations occurring in modern medicine, we have tried to add the pressure of time to our cases. As in real life, we have placed the reader in the middle of complex problems, messy family situations, and a conflicted society. And we have tried to show how medical decisions are confounded by the uncertainty of outcome, whatever decision is made. We think morality is practical, concerned with the impact of the decisions we make on our own and others' lives.

We hope that by going through these exercises conscientiously and pausing to think through and justify the choices, readers will become more empathetic with all participants in the decision-making process and more sensitive to the moral dilemmas they face. We believe thoughtful practice can contribute to becoming a better decision maker, and also a person aware that others with the same information may come to different conclusions. One must then develop tolerance to alternative decisions, but in doing so define the boundaries of one's own tolerance within the range of possible decisions, and in this way decide which are morally acceptable and which are not.

To paraphrase Kant, "Experience without theory is blind. Theory without experience is empty." In this book we have tried to provide readers with both experience (albeit simulated) and some theory, with the opportunity to think about problems, to face them in realistic situations, and then to think about them again with others who can bring scrutiny to bear on the quality of thought.

Baltimore, Maryland
South Bend, Indiana   J. M. F.
June 2000   K. McD.

Contents

CONTENTS

PART II—ADULTHOOD

Chapter 4. Leon, 33

Summary Worsening headaches and confused speech lead Leon's doctor to recommend a brain biopsy. Should Leon and his wife consent?

Issues Informed consent and rational decision making.

Chapter 5. Ms. Williams, 43

Summary A patient chooses the characteristics she wants in her physician.

Issues Paternalism, honesty, and the art of medicine.

Chapter 6 Wanda, 49

Summary A woman with HIV infection is unable and unwilling to control her sexual behavior, posing a threat to the health of many in the community.

Issues Confidentiality, rights of the handicapped, and the politics of disease.

Chapter 7. The Maxistop Study, 59

Summary An Institutional Review Board examines a proposal and consent form for human subjects research.

Issues Risks and benefits of research. Incentives for subjects and investigators. Informed consent. Ethics of placebo trials.

Contents

PART III—CHILDHOOD AND ADOLESCENCE

Chapter 8. Joey, Jessica, Roger, Tom, and Marti, 69

Summary A group of children in a crowded intensive care unit. Space is needed for new patients.

Issues Rights, responsibilities, obligations, and social utility. Conflicts and their interaction with varying medical disorders and prognoses.

Chapter 9. Marti Revisited, 87

Summary Staff on rounds discuss long-term plans for Marti, a quadriplegic 12-year-old, and consider her request to discontinue the respirator.

Issues Autonomy and the depressed adolescent. Rational suicide.

Chapter 10. Tom Revisited, 93

Summary Staff discuss long-range plans for Tom, a child with multiple chronic medical and developmental problems.

Issues Informed consent and fair vs. manipulative presentation of facts. Parental rights and reasonable decision making.

Chapter 11. Billy, 101

Summary An elderly physician schedules a tonsillectomy for a young patient. The treatment may not be needed and the physician has not done the procedure in several years.

Issues Adequate information for patients and families. Physician competence.

Chapter 12. The Castelli Baby, 107

Chapter 13. Christie, 123

PART IV—CONCEPTION AND GESTATION

Chapter 14. The Harrisons' Plans, 149

Chapter 15. The Smyth Saga, 155

Contents

Chapter 16. The Perfect Rexford, 163

Summary   A couple debates what they want for their child and the genetic devices available for producing offspring.

Issues   Genetic manipulation, choosing for others, parental control.

PART V—HEALTH CARE REFORM AND ETHICAL THEORY

Chapter 17. Affordable Health Care, 173

Summary   Advisors review a presidential candidate's speech on health care reform.

Issues   Social justice, social welfare, and individual responsibility. Fairness in the social structure of American health care.

Chapter 18. Ethical Theory and Medical Ethics, 185

A brief presentation of the major theories of medical ethics.

Chapter 19. Making Moral Decisions: A Process Approach, 213

The authors present their approach to making good decisions.

A Note to the Reader

The cases in this book are not meant to be read without pause from beginning to end. Reading straight through would frustrate the whole purpose of the case presentations, which is to place you in the position of a decision maker. We want you to experience some of the uncertainty and tension that surround genuine medical decisions. At the decision points you should stop to ask: "Am I doing the right thing? How can I justify the decision I am making? Is my decision consistent with decisions I have made in other cases? In my own life? Is it appropriate to my role in the case? Have I weighed the relevant factors properly?" Think very carefully at these points, commit yourself to one of the courses of action proposed, then follow the implications of your decision.

PART
I

DEATH AND DYING

chapter

1

* * * * *

Maggie

Margaret Laura O'Sullivan, known to everyone at the home as Maggie, is as lively as one could be at age 84. You are a second-year resident in the family practice program who first met her on rounds with her private physician, Bill Loeb. Dr. Loeb makes rounds once a week at the Hillside Retirement Home to see anyone with a complaint or problem. Between his visits, you are in charge. It is one of the most pleasant rotations of the residency. Things aren't too rushed, no one is very sick, and you have time to get to know the patients—they are your responsibility.

Maggie is a favorite resident at Hillside. The staff loves her because she is not a complainer. A dedicated fan of the Baltimore Orioles, she knows the meaning of adversity and doesn't let mere old age get to her. She can usually be found holding court in "her" corner of the residents' lounge. Always cheerful, usually surrounded by friends, Maggie enjoys life at Hillside; it is her home.

Unlike many of the others, Maggie isn't sick; she has only one prescription medication, to control an erratic heartbeat. You find yourself stopping in the lounge only to ask how she is doing. The answer is always, "Just fine, thank you." Sometimes she brings you up to date on the latest exploits of the Orioles, her "Birds." Often she adds that she is lucky to be better off than poor Mr. So-and-So who had recently been carried off to the hospital.

"No one will ever see him again," she mutters on one occasion, "though it will be a long time before he's dead. You doctors and your infernal machines. Thinking about it is enough to make a body sick. But you know what I want, Doctor. I've told you, and I've told Dr. Loeb. I don't mind taking a few pills now and then, but I do mind nurses and doctors running around pounding on an old lady's chest. And all those machines; I've seen what they can do to a person. That's not what God intended. I don't want any of that resuscitation stuff. When it's my time, I want to go peacefully. The best way to do that, you know, is to keep away from doctors."

"You know," she says on another visit, "did you see the piece in the paper about the family that sued the hospital to get them to turn off the respirator on their mother who had been in a coma for weeks? That's no way to go. What do you think of that Kevorkian fellow? He scares me a little, but some of you doctors don't know when to stop. You just can't let an old lady die in peace."

Another time she says, "My nephew Brian is a lawyer and I've been talking to him about all this resuscitation and machine stuff. I read all about the living will in the paper. I filled out one of them, and I put it in there that if I were resuscitated and kept going, my estate should sue the doctors so they would have to pay for my care while I was on those machines. Brian wasn't sure how some judge might take it, but I put as much stuff as I could on that paper. It's terrible to be hooked up to the darn machines, but then to have to pay for it is too much. I also told Brian that he should try to sue any doctor who did any of that stuff to me. Brian said that he would, and he is a very good lawyer. I am not saying this to threaten you or anything; I'm just telling you how I feel.

"By the way, Doctor, did you read the living will I had them put in my records? I have a copy here in my purse. Here it is. It says right here:"

> If at any time my attending physician certifies in writing that: I have an incurable injury, disease, or illness; my death will occur within a short period of time; and the use of life-prolonging procedures would serve only to prolong the dying process, I direct that such procedures be withheld or withdrawn, and that I be permitted to die naturally. . . .

As she tells the stories of her friends in the home and how they die, it becomes even clearer that her views are well-founded. In light of what she has been saying all along, what happens to Maggie shows the gods' sense of irony.

* * *

When you look over Dr. Loeb's patient list for one of his regular visits to the home, you notice Maggie's name. She had left a note that said, "My ticker doesn't feel right. Would you please stop by and take a listen."

You find Maggie in her room, which is unusual. She is sitting in a lounge chair by the window reading the *Sporting News.* She says that she thinks her heart is skipping beats and is running too fast. You take her pulse, which is 110, and listen to her heart. It does sound irregular.

"Sounds like you found the problem," you tell Maggie. "Your heartbeat is a little off. You probably need some different heart pills. We're going to get an EKG and change your medicine. That ought to take care of it. You'll feel better in a day or two."

When you check in with Dr. Loeb, he says, "Sounds to me like she has an arrhythmia. I'm sure it's nothing much. You should be able to take care of it. Move her down to the infirmary and change her medications. Don't get her all upset with a lot of tests, drawing blood and things. See if you can straighten out the rhythm before it causes her a problem." That afternoon you return to Maggie's room with the portable machine to get an EKG and to reassure her that she'll be fine. They will move her to the infirmary and start her on a new medication in the morning. The same afternoon, you show the EKG to a cardiologist at the hospital who suggests using one of the newer drugs for arrhythmia. She mentions two she has found very effective and suggests you read up on them. That night you read over the literature on both drugs and choose the one that looks most promising for Maggie's problem. The prescribing information recommends that treatment be started with an injection to establish the proper amount of drug in the bloodstream. Afterward, blood levels can be maintained with two to four pills per day. This approach will make Maggie feel better quickly and be good for her morale. Maggie doesn't like the role of sick person.

First thing in the morning, you call the hospital's pharmacy and order the drug delivered to the home's infirmary. You also call the nurses' station and leave a message with the clerk that you will be in later to start Maggie on the new medication. Around 10 A.M., you come through and explain the new medication to Maggie. She is eager to get on with it. While you are sitting at the nurses' station writing the order in her chart, the nurse takes a syringe down the hall to give Maggie the initial injection.

The home's infirmary is a peaceful and quiet place with two nurses and an aide to look after the patients. You are getting up to leave when the nurse comes flying out of Maggie's room. "Call a code on Maggie," she shouts to the nurses' station. You rush into Maggie's room to find her slumped over in bed, the sports pages still clutched in her hand. She has passed out. Her heartbeat is slow, her respiration extremely shallow. Her skin is cold and clammy and has lost all its color. Maggie is having a severe reaction to the medication; she is in shock.

* * *

If this were a TV show, we would pause now for a commercial. Although in real life doctors and nurses do not have time to pause, we can take the luxury of thinking about what should be done for Maggie.

The reflex response, for you have been carefully trained, is to call the code and do everything possible to resuscitate Maggie. But is that what Maggie would want? It is what she would probably want if resuscitation didn't involve any of "those infernal machines." It likely is what she would want if it could quickly return her to her sunny spot as the center of attention in the home's lounge. But what are the chances of this outcome, of recovering and "doing well?"

Wasn't Maggie very clear that she did not want to be resuscitated? She even put it in writing in her living will. But what did she mean when she went on about the "darn machines?" Did that mean she did not want *anything* done? Did she mean she did not want to be placed on a respirator? Not every resuscitation requires a respirator, and even if it does, the machine can be used for a short time or withdrawn if the patient does not do well. Was she really saying that she didn't want to be dependent on anyone or anything for any period of time?

If you think the question of what should be done is settled by Maggie's living will, think again. For all of the status that living wills appear to have, their legal power remains unclear. The law does not tell you whether to resuscitate Maggie. Even in states that recognize living wills and other forms of advance directives, there are not many precedents to guide physicians in ambiguous situations. Few cases have gone far enough in the court system to make plain how such directives should be taken and how much discretion remains for physicians.

If you think that failure to resuscitate Maggie could result in a malpractice claim, realize that resuscitating Maggie could also give rise to a claim, especially if she did poorly. Studies show that court decisions in malpractice cases have little to do with either the quality or the morality of medical care.

Perhaps this event had nothing to do with the medication given, and Maggie's "time had come." But physicians often feel that their treatment has brought about a bad result, and they in turn feel responsible. They therefore feel impelled to attempt to correct the situation.

If this were television, you would see a physician quickly inject the proper antidote and the machine on the wall would show that Maggie's heartbeat had returned to normal. She would then be shown the following morning back in her room, reading the sports pages, feisty as ever. Occasionally this is how things turn out in real life. But resuscitation efforts are often not successful. It may be that considerable time passes before the patient's crisis is discovered and during that time the patient's brain and other organs may be irreparably damaged. Maggie's crisis, however, happened in the infirmary and was immediately recognized. Therefore, her chances of recovery are much better than average.

There are not good statistics on the chances for recovery and on quality of life after a witnessed cardiac event like this, but here are some plausible numbers. Assume that there is about a 70 percent chance that Maggie will do well with no major long-term problems. Also assume that there is a 15 percent chance she will die during or soon after the code. Few will find fault if you resuscitate Maggie and she recovers. If you attempt to resuscitate Maggie and she dies, your decision will not likely be challenged.

But what about the chance (also 15 percent we will assume) that Maggie will survive with substantial brain damage? If she remains in a persistent vegetative state with little or no response to her environment, would Maggie have thought this acceptable? Suppose that she recovers with major problems of speech or memory, or suppose that she has suffered a stroke that paralyzes part of her body; how do you think Maggie would have reacted to those outcomes?

Without subjecting Maggie to this 15 percent risk of bad outcome, how can she enjoy the 85 percent chance of an acceptable outcome—either full recovery or a quick death? The problem facing the decision-maker is the uncertainty and the acceptability of the potential outcomes.

What should you do? Although we are in the midst of a "time-out," real life does not afford that luxury to doctors. In the time you have taken to read these paragraphs, Maggie would probably have died.

*   *   *

- If you decide to play odds and attempt to resuscitate Maggie, how should you justify the decision?
- Does the probability of a good outcome (70 percent chance of recovery) justify ignoring the 15 percent chance of a bad one?
- If the outcome is poor, how will you justify the decision to Brian? To the nursing staff?
- Has Maggie not made her wishes sufficiently plain? Has she really understood enough about what is involved in a resuscitation effort to make a fully informed, autonomous decision to refuse it?
- Are you obliged by the Hippocratic Oath to do everything possible to save Maggie's life?

Pausing as we are doing here is critical because it forces you, the reader, to look into the uncertain outcomes of medical decisions just as physicians must do. When a medical crisis has passed, it is easy to evaluate others' actions in hindsight. When the outcome is uncertain, however, decision-makers must think about many factors. Results, motives, intentions, and circumstances all have a role. It is decision time. What will you do?

Following are two, of many, scenes that could unfold.

Resuscitation I
You quickly lower the bed and begin pumping rhythmically on Maggie's chest. The nurse calls for help and wheels in the infirmary's "crash cart."

Fortunately, she is very experienced with resuscitation and the infirmary is unusually well equipped. The nurse starts an IV line and, at your instruction, begins medications. You listen for stable heart sounds. Nothing yet. You put the heart defibrillation paddles on Maggie's chest and deliver an electrical shock . . . nothing. Two shocks. A third. You listen for the heart rate . . . nothing yet. "Calcium," you say urgently. The nurse pushes the calcium into the IV line and you deliver one more shock. "There, I think that's got it," you say to the nurse. The EKG has returned to a more normal rhythm. "I hope she'll be all right. I hope we got her in time."

"You better have," the nurse responds angrily. "This isn't what Maggie wanted. You know her; she'd rather be dead than an invalid. You want her transferred to the hospital, don't you?"

"Of course," you reply. "I'll call Dr. Loeb and tell him what happened."

As you walk slowly down the hall, you wonder whether you have done right by Maggie. Is this what Maggie wanted? Was there any choice but to do everything you could, everything you had long trained to do? Maggie wanted to be alive and vital. Will she be that? Above all, she did not want a lingering time of incapacity. Is that what you have created?

Resuscitation II

As you are cranking down Maggie's bed, all her conversations about the kind of care she did not want come back in a flash. You turn to the nurse and say, "This isn't what Maggie would want. We'll give it a quick shot. If we can't get her heart rhythm back right away, we'll quit."

You begin pumping rhythmically on Maggie's chest. The nurse calls for help and wheels in the infirmary's crash cart. Fortunately, she is very experienced with resuscitation and the infirmary is unusually well equipped. The nurse starts an IV line and, at your instruction, begins medications. You listen for stable heart sounds. Nothing yet. You put the paddles on Maggie's chest . . . Nothing . . . two shocks, and you listen again.

"That's all," you say. "No good. At least we gave it a shot. If she's not back by now, things probably wouldn't go well for her anyway."

As you walk slowly down the hall, you wonder whether you have done right by Maggie. Is this what Maggie wanted? At least there was now no chance Maggie would have the lingering debilitation she most feared. If she had been younger, of course, you would have worked much longer. But you never know about these things.

* * *

The difference between these two scenarios is slight—only one more medication and one more shock and the heart resumed its rhythm. Without that extra effort, Maggie is dead. How do you feel about that? Is there an ethical dimension to deciding when enough is enough?

There are many possible endings to this story; outcomes in medicine are rarely certain. The chances that Maggie could survive without a full resuscitation effort are vanishingly small. What will be the outcome of the resuscitation described in the first scene? We have written out two of the possibilities. Since both are possible outcomes of the same efforts on your part, you cannot choose the one you prefer. Flip a coin to see how things turn out. Heads points to outcome number one; tails, to number two.

Outcome 1

The day after the resuscitation, Maggie is sitting up in her hospital bed having breakfast when you and Dr. Loeb come by on rounds. Brian is there and greets both of you warmly. "Good work, Doctor. I hear you did a great job. We're all so grateful to have Aunt Maggie with us. We've been told that she was only a hair's breadth from death, and you brought her back."

"God bless you, Doctor," Maggie chimes in. "But when can I get out of this dreadful place? Can I go back to the home tomorrow?"

Dr. Loeb puts his hand on Maggie's. "You're a tough old lady, Maggie. That ticker of yours has miles to go; it just stumbled for a minute."

In the hall, you talk with Dr. Loeb about your doubts about resuscitating Maggie. "Would you have resuscitated her, Bill? Should I have said something to the nurse about a DNR (do not resuscitate) order?"

"You did a good job. Of course that was the right thing to do. Look at Maggie. If you hadn't done it, she wouldn't be with us now."

Outcome 2

When you enter Maggie's room with Dr. Loeb early the next morning, Brian is already there. Maggie is pale and her straggly gray hair frames a face that has aged many years. The oxygen mask covers her mouth and nose, and she burbles a bit with each breath. Maggie is alive, but the old Maggie is not there, at least not yet. Will she ever be?

"Maggie!" Dr. Loeb shouts. "Maggie, can you hear me?" He pats her face a little bit. "Maggie!" One eye opens partially. He senses more than hears her attempt to say, "What?"

Dr. Loeb turns to Brian, "It doesn't look good, Brian, but it's hard to tell yet. I think she'll make it, but I don't know if we'll have the old Maggie back. Despite the fine efforts of my young colleague here, her brain may have been without enough oxygen for too long. Or she may have had a stroke during that episode. At her age, the brain doesn't have the reserve a younger person's might have. I know Maggie didn't want to be on machines and she didn't want to be in this state. We put her on a respirator for only a few hours. We've now taken her off the machine; what you see is only a little extra oxygen. If that's still okay with you, we won't do anything heroic. We'll keep her comfortable and give her whatever medicine is necessary, hoping she can get back to being herself."

"Thanks a lot," Brian glowers. "She told you two very clearly that she didn't want to be resuscitated, and you went ahead and did it anyway. All she wanted was to go peacefully, and look what you've done. This isn't Aunt Maggie and this isn't what she wanted. She told you! She emphasized that she wanted to die peacefully. Everyone at the home knew it. Why did you resuscitate her? Now you tell me that you won't put her on machines. You damn well better not put her on machines. But it's too late; you've already got her in the state she dreaded most.

"I know she threatened that I would sue you and sue the hospital for the bills and all that stuff. I could do that, you know. But that's not going to help Aunt Maggie. Please, please, just let her go peacefully. That's all she wanted."

*   *   *

Do not take your position as an armchair physician too easily. Practicing physicians must deal with issues like this all the time. What was the right thing to do back when the nurse first called the code on Maggie? Does the moral quality of the decision rest on the outcome? If so, then how can physicians make appropriate moral and clinical decisions if they are judged by unforeseeable results? Are physicians always forced to look backward to find the moral character of what they have done? What reasons would you advance for resuscitating or not resuscitating Maggie?

Do you know what your mother, father, aunt, or brother would want in such a situation? Have you discussed it with them? How would you, or they, ensure that the physician acted in accordance with their wishes in a situation such as Maggie's?

chapter

2

* * * * *

Jill

Jill looks fine sitting there in front of you. She is in her late 40s, slender and attractive. She had first seen you five years ago when her company had signed their employees up with your HMO. Two years ago her gynecologist had sent a note telling you that Jill had been referred to the group's oncologist for a suspicious lump detected on a mammogram. As Jill's primary care physician, you were expected to direct her path through the HMO's system of referrals and consultants.

After the biopsy, Jill agreed to a vigorous approach to what appeared to be an aggressive tumor. She underwent radical surgery and endured many of its complications. The chemotherapy and radiation had made her violently ill for months, and she appeared to have aged at least ten years during that time. Although not involved in her day-to-day care, you had often seen her in the hospital and checked on her progress throughout this ordeal. As far as you could tell, her care had been excellent, state-of-the-art, and Jill seemed to have done very well.

When Jill comes to see you this time, she looks as if she had something else on her mind.

"Yesterday I spoke with my oncologist. She gave me the results of last week's scan and, as I feared, there are metastases. They must be the cause for my recent headaches and the weakness in my arm. She suggested that we do more radiation and another round of chemotherapy while we search for a bone marrow donor and plan for a bone marrow transplant.

"I've been through torture once, and what she is planning is even worse. The oncologist says that, even with the latest chemotherapies, the numbers for my kind of cancer are not good. I'm tired. I'm sick of fighting. I think I've finally gotten to the point where I can see I'm going to lose, and I accept that."

You respond that you understand. It certainly has been a tough two years, and Jill has borne it amazingly well. There are still lots of new things that can be done, and new, more powerful combinations of drugs that can be used.

"You need to *listen*, Doctor," Jill replies. "I'm saying that I'm tired of this struggle. I know your doctor tricks—all those things about maintaining the patient's hope. We talk about them all the time in the support groups. I haven't lost hope. I'm just being realistic, hoping for a calm and peaceful death. Is there anything wrong with that?

"You know, some of the women in those support groups are just fantastic. They have the most amazing courage and determination to beat this dreadful disease. I really admire them. But there are others who just can't be realistic, who never face the facts or the odds. I don't want to be like them. I've had plenty of time to think about it, and I decided that if my cancer recurred I would plan for my death. I want it to be a good death, and I want it to occur when the time is right. I want you to help me.

"You have really been very helpful through these trying times. I'm depending on you. I have no family to speak of. My brother lives in California, but we've never been close. My dad died a long time ago, and Mom died last year after nearly three months in the hospital. I certainly don't want to go like her. It was horrible. She didn't know who I was; she didn't know who she was. She had no control over any aspect of her life. I don't ever want to be in that situation.

"I think I could probably live with another round of therapy if the cancer had gone to my bones. I have a high tolerance for pain. But with metastases to the brain, I'm going to lose control sooner or later, and that is what I fear the most. That is why I am turning to you now, while I am competent. I want your help. In the groups we've talked about others who had arrived at the point where they wanted to stop, but their doctor said they were too depressed or not competent to make that decision. Others were just too physically disabled to end their own lives and were forced to continue suffering, especially the awful indignities of incompetence, incontinence, and loss of control. I never want to be like them."

You suggest that Jill is depressed. Perhaps this is the normal reaction to her predicament.

"Yes, of course I'm depressed; any normal person in my situation would be. The past two years have been rough, and that report wasn't any fun to hear. But I've been a long time coming to this decision. I'm still very competent. I work full time, in charge of planning the redevelopment of inner-city Bridgeport. My work is going exceptionally well at the moment. Depression is not interfering with any of my other judgments, so it makes me uneasy when you suggest it's interfering with this one.

"The other women said that the usual trick is to send patients who want to quit treatment to a psychiatrist to determine if they are depressed. The psychiatrist finds that they are depressed and starts medication. There are plenty of new medications. They are prescribed one after the other, and each takes several weeks to see whether it works. In the meantime women are forced to continue treatment as their disease progresses. Shrinks never consider that perhaps the depression is a realistic reaction to the situation and is fully rational. They think this sort of depression is some isolated disease and therefore treatable.

"I want you to help me. I want a good death at the proper time. That is my goal. I'm a planner; both professionally and personally I set goals and make plans for achieving them.

"I need you to help me plan the when and the how of this good death. I know that euthanasia is legal in Holland, but uprooting myself to move there is unrealistic. Assisted suicide is legal in Oregon, but I would have to set up residency and find a physician willing to get to know me and my personality and problems. If I moved, I would have to give up my job, which I love and which I plan to continue as long as I'm able.

"I've read a lot of stuff about living wills and advanced directives, all the items from your pamphlet rack, and more besides. But none of those things goes far enough for me. The living will law in this state only applies when I am dying, and I don't want things to get to that point. So far as a health care representative or someone who has durable power of attorney for health care, I am not close enough to anyone to hand over that power.

"People often consider discontinuing therapy, turning off machines, and such passive moves as a way of hastening death, or at least not prolonging illness. I need to go further than that. Discontinuing therapy only allows someone to suffer while dying of the complications. I want to specify in advance a set of circumstances under which you would provide me with a lethal amount of medication that I could take, and help me to decide on the proper time to take it. Or, if I'm not able to do it myself, I want you to promise to give me a lethal injection.

"I am a very independent person. I find it very hard to ask others for help. But will *you* help me? Please?"

*   *   *

You are now on the spot. This thoroughly sensible person is putting a reasonable proposition before you. There are a number of possible responses.

You Could Reject Jill's Request Outright

You may believe absolutely that "thou shalt not kill," that no individual should directly and intentionally take the life of another. Agreeing with Jill's request would be agreeing to direct an intentional killing.

If your refusal is based on religious grounds, how should Jill relate to your views since she does not have any particular religious convictions? How would you answer someone who accused you of imposing your views and beliefs on your patient?

If your refusal is based on legal grounds, would you acquiesce to Jill's request if the law in your state allowed physician-assisted suicide? Does the law place a moral restriction on your actions, or does its only power come from the penalties it can impose? You could avoid those problems by helping Jill in a way that your action could not be detected. Is it acceptable to violate the law if you are sure you will not be caught? Even if your action were detected and a prosecutor took the case to a jury, it is unlikely that you would be convicted. Does the absence of bad consequences mean your action is morally acceptable?

Do you as a physician have rights *not* to participate in actions that you find objectionable? Remember that Jill chose you because of your caring, compassionate relationships with your patients. Why should your compassion not extend to relieving her suffering?

You Could Acquiesce to Jill's Request

You might respond, "Yes, I'll help you when the time comes." Does this statement commit you to appear, on Jill's demand, with a syringe full of the lethal medication?

Is there a middle ground that would ease your conscience? As a physician you would, of course, prescribe enough medicine (e.g., morphine) so that the individual would feel little pain. If you gave just enough morphine to mitigate the pain, and then just a little bit more, the individual might stop breathing and would no longer suffer. Is there a clear distinction in this case between killing and letting die? Is the distinction in the mind of the physician or is it apparent from what the physician does? Are people clear about their intentions in such difficult situations?

Some have tried to sharpen the distinction between killing and letting die by employing a "principle of double effect." This principle is more fully explained in Chapter 18. Briefly, the principle holds that while an evil effect (in this case, the hastened death of a patient) of an action may be foreseen, that does not mean the evil effect is intended. On this theory, physicians may justifiably use morphine to ease pain so long as they do not intend to bring about the patient's death. Does this principle help you more clearly think through Jill's situation?

Is There a Third Alternative, Not Everything Jill Wants, but Close?

Suppose Jill had asked you for some sleeping pills to help her at night during these difficult times. Would you tell her to take two at night, but not to take 42 pills because they might be lethal? Would you only give her 10 at a time to make it harder to take a lethal dose? Would you give her 100 at a time and leave those decisions to her? If you take this approach, can you absolve yourself from having any intentions at all about the way Jill uses the prescribed medication?

Before deciding on your final response to Jill's request, review the ethical considerations that follow.

Patient Autonomy.   Whose life is it, anyway? The principle of patient autonomy is simple—the patient makes decisions about her own life. If medical practice is built on patient autonomy, are patients the sole *moral* agents in deciding the course of their medical care? Other than professional responsibility for competent treatment, what moral stake do physicians have in medical care? Without such a stake, what is the basis for either agreeing with or refusing Jill's request?

Utilitarianism.   Utilitarianism requires that we look at the consequences of physician-assisted suicide for the roles and responsibilities of physicians. One potential social consequence of accepting physician-assisted suicide is that the public would lose trust in physicians and confidence that they were always working for their patients' good. When another patient in Jill's predicament goes to her HMO physician, how can she be confident that her doctor is not agreeing with her request solely to avoid the future costs of her illness? If physicians bring death as well as life and healing, would people lose trust and fail to seek help when they should? On the other hand, it is possible that allowing physicians to help their patients avoid suffering and even to assist in achieving a good death could increase faith that the physician is working for the best interest of the patient. Which is the more likely consequence of legalizing physician-assisted suicide?

Social Role of Medicine.   Does the financial power and social prestige of medicine substantially diminish patient autonomy in assisted suicide situations? If physicians agree to requests like Jill's, will they raise administered death as an option even when patients do not bring it up themselves? Would the very suggestion push some patients, perhaps the elderly or the borderline depressed, toward that choice? Can you make an agreement with Jill and not allow it to affect the social role of medicine? Is this the start down some slippery slope toward euthanasia for the willing, and finally perhaps for the not-so-willing? Would euthanasia give patients freedom to consent to an additional procedure, or would freedom be reduced because patients might be pressured—by family, society, physicians, insurers—to accept a quick death?

Quality Care at the End of Life.   Would an agreement with Jill reinforce the "quick fix" style of American medicine and weaken the moral commitment to care at the end of life? If Jill wants to die at the start of her last crisis, what will you say to those who want to die at the beginning of the next-to-last crisis, or even the first crisis? Would physician-assisted suicide lead to a loss of moral fiber reducing people's resolve to live and fight disease?

Killing versus Letting Die. What are the moral implications for medical practice if accepting physician-assisted suicide means abandoning the distinction between killing and letting die? Much of the resistance to physician assisted suicide and euthanasia rests on maintaining this distinction. In the case of severely ill patients, does this distinction have any weight? When Jill is dying, does it make a difference whether the physician gives her morphine before removing the ventilator and letting her breathe for a while, or giving more morphine and ending life a little sooner? If this distinction disappeared, would physicians who reject killing feel compelled to continue aggressive treatment, doing anything they can to keep patients from dying?

Procedural Safeguards. Should you act without accepted procedures in place? In the United States, with the exception of Oregon, there are no protections or procedures for carrying out euthanasia. Administrative procedures could be obstructive headaches. On the other hand, they may protect society against "lone rangers" who choose to act without sufficient safeguards for patient autonomy and careful control.

Resolution
Tell Jill you need to think about it. Write a first prescription for an antidepressant and make an appointment to see her in two weeks to check on side effects. Promise her an answer then; it would not be fair to stall longer if she will have to find another physician. As you think through your response, take time to think about some of the alternative responses you might make, and consider their consequences.

Think about your role as a physician. Would it change the moral situation if you were Jill's friend instead of her doctor, and she asked this of you?

chapter
3
* * * * *

Ed Martinez

"Mrs. Martinez, . . . Marta," you call out as you walk into the waiting room outside the operating suite. Marta Martinez, sitting in the far corner of the room waiting for her husband to come out of surgery, looks up from her magazine. "We have to talk. Let's go to the conference room across the hall." Marta Martinez is in her mid-50s, a nurse's aid at Community Hospital. You have known Marta and Eduardo for years in their various jobs in the hospital and around town. Ed put the roof on your lake cottage two or three years ago. This is not going to be an easy discussion.

Ed Martinez is a 55-year-old who has a small construction business in town. You are a general surgeon at Community. Ed is a healthy specimen, admitted now for removal of a gallstone. You have been this family's surgeon before, luckily being there for Ed's emergency appendectomy and referring Marta elsewhere for a consultation before ultimately doing a lumpectomy when most of the other surgeons in the area would have done a radical mastectomy.

Everything seemed to be going well in the operating room when you noticed that Ed's tissues were turning blue. Checking with the anesthesiologist, a new man you had not worked with often, you found that something was wrong. The anesthesiologist worked rapidly with his machines, but Ed's blood pressure had dropped precipitously, and a quick listen with the stethoscope revealed a cardiac arrest. The anesthesiologist administered stimulants while you ordered and used the defibrillator. You had no idea of the cause of the problem. Had the anesthesia tube dislodged? Although it seemed like an eternity, it took perhaps four or five minutes, maybe more, to get Ed's heart going again. Had there been enough oxygen to maintain the brain during that time? Would he recover? Would he be impaired? If so, how great would the damage be? The outcome is not at all clear at this point. The session with Marta is going to be very painful.

"What's the matter?" asks Marta as you walk into the conference room. "Is

Eduardo okay? Didn't things go well?" From the look on your face, Marta can tell there has been trouble.

"Sit down, Marta," you say, "we've got a real problem. I am not entirely sure that I know what happened, but there must have been a problem with the anesthesia. Ed's heart stopped on the table. We got it going again. The brain can only stand three or four minutes without oxygen, and we can't be exactly sure how much, if any, brain damage occurred. It could be considerable.

"In the last few minutes I've been thinking about what Ed said as we stood by the cottage, admiring the roof he had just finished and talking about this and that. He said that he'd never want to just cling to life, hooked to a machine. He would never want to be dependent or a burden. Ed was much too vigorous and self-sufficient for that. Well, everything he feared is a real possibility now.

"It's possible, of course, that Ed's brain and heart suffered such a severe insult that he won't make it no matter what we do. But I don't think the cardiac arrest lasted that long. It's also possible, on the other side, that we caught all this in time and that Ed will come out with little or no damage. That's not likely either. I'm afraid the biggest chance is for something in between, that Ed's brain will be impaired, perhaps even severely impaired. If it is severely impaired, he might not be able to talk, to care for himself, or even to think. He could survive for weeks, even years, in such a state. I just don't know."

There is a terrible pause as Marta sobs quietly.

"Isn't there any hope?" she asks. "Can't you do anything? I love him so much, but I don't want him to suffer. Why did this have to happen? He is such a good man and a good husband. Isn't there any hope?"

You put your arm around Marta's shoulder. "There is hope, Marta, but not very much, and we may pay a tremendous price for it. They're finishing up now in the OR. We'll send him to the ICU and keep him on a respirator; there's a very good chance that he'll survive, but there's also a great risk he'll be substantially impaired. If we disconnect him now, we know he won't survive. But that's not realistic. Treatment in the ICU is the standard of care. I have no choice but to send him there."

*　*　*

Should this standard of practice be changed? If, in the course of surgery, it appears that the patient's brain has been severely damaged—whether by an accident of anesthesia or surgery or by a complication that could not be anticipated—should the anesthesia equipment be turned off on the spot with the certainty that the patient will die? Or should every patient be given the chance to recover, even if that means many patients will linger on in a vegetative state while only a few survive nearly intact? What ethical issues would be involved in such a change, for example, what additional information would patients need before surgery and how could the risks and benefits of resuscitation be adequately explained? How might a change in policy affect patients' attitudes toward surgery?

Ed Goes to the ICU

You stop in the recovery room to check with the nurse. Ed seems to be stable, but there is no way of knowing how much damage has been done. The anesthesia is wearing off, but Ed is not yet breathing on his own and continues to require a respirator. Despite your concern for him and his wife, you follow the standard procedure and write the admission note for the ICU.

After watching the gurney disappear down the hall, you return to the conference room to talk with Marta.

"Ed is in the ICU now; you can see him there in an hour or so. We'll do everything we can to support him now. Tomorrow we'll do an electroencephalogram (EEG), a test of his brain waves. That may give us some clues about his recovery, but the clinical signs are more important. Most people who are going to recover will show a dramatic response in two or three days. If Ed is not doing well and the EEG shows extensive damage, we can consider turning off the respirator.

"Don't be frightened by all the equipment around his bed: the respirator, cardiac monitors, IV lines, and catheters. They're all part of standard care in that unit. There is nothing to do now but hope and pray."

Three Days Later

It is now three long days since the operation. Ed Martinez remains on a respirator, not able to breathe on his own. His blood pressure and heart rate are normal. Responding only to intense pain, he is deeply comatose. Yesterday's EEG showed evidence of severe brain dysfunction. Because there is some brain activity, Ed is not brain dead, but he has not shown the dramatic response for which you and Marta were hoping.

You spot Marta as you leave the ICU. She looks fatigued and depressed. You have been talking to her once or twice a day, trying to keep up her hope. Now it is time to face it. You take her and one of the ICU nurses to a nearby conference room.

"Marta," you begin, "things look very bad. Ed shows no sign of waking up. I'm afraid our worst fears are coming true. It's now clear that he has suffered severe and permanent brain injury. Patients who are going to make a good recovery virtually all show some positive response by now. Ed is hardly responsive at all. The EEG confirms that he suffered severe damage, and the finding confirms our clinical exam. But Ed does not meet the established criteria for brain death. I don't know how long he could go on like this, but with good nursing care and the respirator, it could be a long time: weeks, months, or even years. This is the state he was most afraid of and did not want. All we're doing now with our high-technology medicine is prolonging his dying, and he enjoys no reasonable life in the meantime.

"It may be time for us to stop, time to turn off the respirator. Since Ed requires the machine to breathe, stopping it would be a merciful way of allowing him to die. Many people say that this is not killing him, but merely removing the technology that is artificially preserving his life. While some patients in Ed's condition live on in a vegetative state, it's exceedingly unlikely that he would return to anything like normal human function. What do you think we should do?"

"I don't know," replies Marta. "I love him so much that even just sitting by his bedside is a great comfort to me. I can't bear to think of life without him, but I know how he felt about this. He wouldn't want to be kept alive in this state. He wouldn't want to be a burden, although I certainly don't find him one.

"But isn't this covered in Mr. Martinez's living will?" asked the nurse. "It's in the chart. He filled one out when he came in for the surgery."

"I've read it," you respond, "but I don't think it's of much use. It is the standard form we use in this state. When the admitting nurse asked Ed about advance directives, she was following the requirements of the Patient Self-Determination Act. According to her note in Ed's chart, he filled out a living will but didn't appoint a health care representative or give anyone a durable power of attorney for his health care."

"Oh, I don't know anything about all those details," Marta replies. "Eduardo always handled those things. He thought the living will was all we needed."

"The paper is right here in the chart," you respond. "Let's look it over to see if it applies to his situation now:"

> If at any time I have an incurable injury, disease, or illness certified in writing to be a terminal condition by my attending physician, and my attending physician has determined that my death will occur within a short period of time, and the use of life prolonging procedures would only serve to artificially prolong the dying process, I direct that such procedures be withheld or withdrawn, and that I be permitted to die naturally . . .
>
> (From the *Indiana Code* 16-36-4-10)

"It's not clear that Ed's case is covered. The living will in this state, like many of them, was written for patients who die slow deaths from chronic diseases such as cancer. It does not take good account of people who suffer from a sudden catastrophe.

"There's another document that might be more to the point. Marta, did Ed sign an organ donor card? There is sometimes a record of it on his driver's license."

"Yes," said Marta, "he did sign the card. Ed was big on that sort of thing every time they had a special on TV about it. He always used to joke, 'Parts is parts,' he'd say. But how does that come up now? I thought that was for young people who fell off their motorcycles."

"Well," you reply, "the rules are changed. Or better, we're going back to the old rules, before brain death was accepted. We're again looking at cardiac death. Surgeons can remove organs a few minutes after the heart stops. Even someone of Ed's age still has some good time left on many of his organs."

"The only thing I can think of," Marta says, "is to tell you to do what you think best. We've always thought of you as our friend, not just our doctor."

"If you're willing to consider taking Ed off the respirator, then you probably should talk to the transplant people and hear what they have to say."

"Actually, I have to stop here. As Ed's doctor, my job is to do what's best for him. I know it sounds silly, but to avoid even the appearance of conflict of interest I have to get someone from the Transplant Resource Center to explain the procedure to you. You should hear the proposal from them. I'll page them to come over."

The Transplant Team's Presentation

"Good morning, Mrs. Martinez. I'm Sandi Stanislas, a family advocate at the hospital. My job is to insure that you get the emotional support you need in this difficult situation and to be sure that you're not pressured to do something you might regret later. Let me introduce Dr. George Roberts, a surgeon from the Regional Transplant Center, and our transplant nurse Jennifer Chen. I'm sorry we're meeting under such sad circumstances."

"Let me say that we've already looked at your husband's chart," began Ms. Chen, "and determined that he would be a helpful donor. Several of his vital organs, especially his liver, are almost certainly in a condition that they could be life saving for other people. My colleague Dr. Roberts will explain the procedure."

"I assume that your doctor has already explained that your husband has sustained severe brain damage. He's very unlikely to recover consciousness. The 'best' we can hope for, and I put the word in quotes, is that your husband would linger in a permanent vegetative state. You're thinking about taking him off the respirator to let him die in peace. The most probable scenario is that his physician will remove the respirator and he will quickly die. He may linger for a short time, but his brain is so damaged that he will soon stop breathing and pass on. Of course, his doctor will give him some sedatives to make absolutely sure he does not suffer.

"Instead of carrying out this procedure in the ICU, your doctor can do it in an operating room. You can be there, if you'd like. We'll prep your husband as if we were going to do some surgery. Then the physician will disconnect him, and he will die peacefully. We'll ask you to leave as soon as he draws his last breath. Five minutes after his heart stops beating, we'll certify his death and start the process of taking his organs. Our procedures are compatible with any of the usual funeral customs. While we can't guarantee that your husband's organs will be suitable for transplant, I am confident you will have the consolation that your husband was able to help others in death much as I imagine he did in life."

"Do you have any questions, Mrs. Martinez?" asks Sandi. "I am sorry to bring in new faces at this point. We know you're comfortable with your own doctor, but we need to be completely sure that you don't feel pressured in any way, and that this decision is completely your own."

*　*　*

Now you must work with Marta to make a decision. At this point, postponing the decision to take Ed off the respirator is as much a decision as any other, and it probably eliminates the possibility of using his organs for transplant. Think very carefully, because this decision may be irrevocable.

For the purposes of this discussion, assume that Marta will accept whatever recommendation you make.

If you decide to turn off the respirator, consider the justification for your decision:

- Is it justified by Ed's wishes even if only verbally expressed? Does turning off the respirator respect Eduardo Martinez's autonomy? How certain are you that this is what he wants?
- Is it justified by Marta's acquiescence? Is Marta expressing Ed's view, or is she acting as a surrogate, trying to do what's best for him?
- Is it justified by what is in Ed's best interest? How is it in his interest to be dead?
- Is disconnecting Ed in the best interests of Marta, their insurance company, the hospital, or society? Are any of these considerations morally legitimate?

The possibility of organ donation adds another set of moral complexities. While the decision to disconnect someone from a respirator can be separated intellectually from the decision to transplant his organs, it cannot be separated in a family's emotions. You need to consider several ethical issues about the way the transplant team approached this issue with Marta and the process of transplantation itself:

- Once the issue of transplantation is raised, can we be sure that anyone involved is acting solely on the patient's behalf and not on the part of those who will benefit from the organ transplants?
- Does it insure Marta's moral autonomy that the transplant team make its presentation to Marta without Ed's physician present, especially since, in this case, Marta is relying on that physician for personal and emotional support?
- When the transplant team talks about sedation to be sure Ed feels no pain, are they really talking about suppressing his breathing to insure that he dies? What precautions should be taken to insure that all are acting according to Ed's wishes or in his best interests?
- Once it is established that someone is irreversibly and severely brain damaged, would it be morally acceptable to stop treating the individual as a human person and to deal with him or her as a source of organs? Are all the precautions about taking organs only after the person is surely dead only a foolish rationalization?

After thinking about these factors, if you still want to turn off the respirator but don't recommend organ donation, read the following section. If you decide to turn off the respirator and get the organ donation, skip ahead to "The Organ Donation." If you decide to leave Ed on the respirator and review the situation in several weeks, go to "Two Weeks Later."

You Turn Off the Respirator

Marta comes to be with Ed when he dies. She holds his hand while you turn off the respirator. As you both stand there, Ed Martinez does not breathe. He turns a little blue, and his heart rate drops to 70, then to 60. After three minutes it goes to 50, then 40. He takes a big gasping breath, and his heartbeat increases to 55. Thirty seconds later he takes another gasping breath, followed by several more. Then he begins to breathe on his own. Damn! His heart rate returns to normal and his breathing becomes regular. You predicted that it was only your machine that was keeping him alive, but you were wrong.

You and Marta both walk out of the ICU and speechlessly enter a conference room. You sit down together, but neither of you say anything for a long time.

"I just don't know what to do, Marta. I don't know what to say. We'll just see how it goes for the next week or so." Then you help the sobbing woman to her car.

Turn to "Six Weeks Later."

The Organ Donation

The next day, Marta meets with you in the ICU. She is plainly drained emotionally.

"I can't think about anything else," she starts. "Ed has been my whole life. But now it's time to pass on some of that life. That hope means so much to me. I'm coming to grips with the fact that Ed is gone. But it really helps me when I think that he'll help someone else live on. This organ transplant now means everything to me.

"Also, I want to be there at the end. Please set it up so I can go to the operating room when you disconnect the machine. That nice lady Sandi can take me away as soon as Ed stops breathing, and then you can get on with what you have to do."

You assure her that the arrangements will be made for the next day, and leave Marta in the ICU holding Ed's hand.

Early the next morning, you join Marta in the ICU and walk with her as the staff wheels Ed, still connected to the respirator, to the operating room. The transplant team checks in and assures you that they are ready to go. Marta holds Ed's hand while you turn off the respirator. As you both stand there, Ed Martinez does not breathe. He turns a little blue, and his heart rate drops to 70, then to 60. After three minutes it goes to 50, then 40. He takes a big gasping breath, and his heartbeat increases to 55. Thirty seconds later he takes another breath, followed by several more. Then he begins to breathe on his own. Damn! His heart rate returns to normal and his breathing becomes regular. You predicted that it was only your machine that was keeping him alive, but you were wrong.

You and Marta both walk out of the operating room and speechlessly enter a conference room. You sit down together, but neither of you say anything for a long time.

"I just don't know what to do, Marta. I don't know what to say. We'll just see how it goes for the next week or so." Then you help the sobbing woman to her car.

Turn to "Six Weeks Later."

Two Weeks Later

It's now two weeks since the original surgery, and Ed continues to rest comfortably in the ICU. He remains on the respirator and is fed intravenously. The neurologist has written in the chart that he is in a persistent vegetative state. He still doesn't breathe on his own and remains deeply comatose. The EEG shows a low level of abnormal activity.

Marta sits down in your office for another of what have become increasingly awful discussions.

"Marta," you begin, "last night I spoke again with Bill Baldwin, chairman of the Ethics Committee, and he agrees that now we can turn off the respirator. Although Ed isn't brain dead, he's more like Karen Ann Quinlan—although it's too soon to say his vegetative state is permanent, we can now say it is persistent. And the chance of his waking up from the kind of injury he's suffered is slim to none. Bill thinks we'd be legally and morally in the clear. Is that okay with you?"

"Maybe you should have done it in the operating room," Marta responds. "These few weeks have been the most terrible of my life. I don't know if he's suffered as much as I have. Perhaps he can't feel anything; but if he knew, he would be suffering. It's time for all of this to be over."

Marta comes into the ICU to be with Ed when he dies. She holds his hand while you turn off the respirator. As you stand there, Ed does not breathe. He turns a little blue, and his heart rate drops to 70, then to 60. After three minutes it goes to 50, then 40. He takes a big gasping breath, and his heartbeat increases to 55. Thirty seconds later he takes another breath, followed by several more. Then he begins to breathe on his own. Damn! His heart rate returns to normal and his breathing becomes regular. You predicted that it was only your machine that was keeping him alive, but you were wrong.

You and Marta walk out of the ICU together and speechlessly enter a conference room. You both sit down, but neither of you say anything for a long time.

"I just don't know what to do, Marta. I don't know what to say. We'll just see how it goes." Then you help the sobbing woman to her car.

Six Weeks Later

You call Marta to your office for a conference. "About the only option left to us is to discontinue feeding Ed. He is not on the respirator any more; he's breathing on his own. Ed could linger, unless he's lucky enough to develop some fatal complications. There are two possibilities at this point: we can put a permanent tube in his stomach [a gastrostomy tube or "g-tube"] and send him off to a nursing home that's prepared to care for this kind of patient. Or we can stop feeding him here. If we take out the nasogastric tube [a tube through the nose to the stomach, "ng-tube"] and stop the feeding, we'll be depriving him of fluids and nutrition. It might take two weeks or so for him to die if we do that but, since he's comatose, there shouldn't be any pain or suffering. If you try to get the nursing home to discontinue the feeding, it will be much more complicated than doing it here in the hospital.

"But I have to tell you, Marta, that we need to come to a decision on this. Ed spent two weeks in the ICU and four on a regular unit. Your insurance company and the hospital's utilization committee are demanding that we justify this level of care. Frankly, we're not doing enough for Ed to keep him here. Also, your resources have got to be running low since you have to pay 20 percent of the bill.

"The Nancy Cruzan case, maybe you read about it, has set the boundaries for handling this kind of situation. Nancy Cruzan, a young Missouri woman, was in an auto accident that left her unconscious and unresponsive. Her parents decided that Nancy wouldn't have wanted to live on in that condition. They requested that the rehabilitation hospital stop her feedings, but the hospital refused to do so without a court order. The case ended up going to the U.S. Supreme Court. Although there were a lot of legal technicalities involved, that Court did lay down a basic guideline that is pretty well accepted.

"After reviewing a number of previous decisions from Karen Quinlan to Claire Conroy, the court concluded that hydration and nutrition, food and fluids to everyone else, are medical care. The Court said, 'we assume the U.S. Constitution would grant a competent person a constitutionally protected right to refuse lifesaving hydration and nutrition' [*Cruzan v. Director, Missouri Department of Health,* 1990]. Most of the decision actually dealt with the legal technicalities of how people might refuse such treatment.

"The result of the decision is to allow each state to set its own standards. Missouri set a high standard of evidence, and the Supreme Court accepted that. But other states could accept different standards. Following state court decisions, New Jersey and New York have very complex procedures. The practice in this state is a little easier. Even though you are not Ed's legally appointed guardian for health care, as his wife you can request that we stop the feeding. The hospital has to be convinced that you are acting in good faith, which means you're not trying to profit from Ed's death. Also, the hospital has to be convinced that Ed would not want to be kept alive in his present condition. I don't think I'll have any trouble convincing the Ethics Committee that Ed would want the feeding stopped.

"I know this is something of a long way around, but you need to know that we could stop feeding Ed. What do you think?"

"Well," Marta says, "I don't know about all those procedures lawyers worry about, but it just doesn't feel the same to take the food and water away from him. Eduardo so loved the meals I cooked; food and our family dishes meant so much to him. I mean, respirators are ugly machines with tubes hanging all over them. But in the hospital I work with stomach tubes all the time. A gastrostomy tube is the most ordinary thing in the world. How can we take that away from him? Even though he can't feel it, how can we take away his nourishment? How can we let him die of thirst?

"I know you've always done what you thought best and I've always thought you've had Eduardo's interests at heart. I know that it's just a wife's emotion, but taking away his food and water just doesn't feel right to me."

* * *

How will you respond to Marta? Is taking away food and water provided by a nasogastric tube the same as taking away a respirator? Remember that taking away a respirator takes away the air we breathe. Is there a distinction between killing Ed and letting him die? When you removed the respirator, he breathed on his own. But if you take away the nasogastric tube, he cannot eat on his own. Removing that tube will surely result in his death. Is that different from killing him? Can you make a distinction between killing him and stopping "extraordinary" or "heroic" care, even though you recognize that he will die after you stopped therapy? Is feeding through a tube ordinary or extraordinary care? Who is the hero of heroic care?

If stopping care is not different from killing him, why not do just that? Why should it take a week or more to let him die, inefficiently, even painfully to those who watch, when that result could be achieved in minutes?

How should you go about making this decision? Marta is reluctant, but doubtless could be brought around. How hard should you work at persuading her? Does trying to persuade her mean that you are exerting undue pressure? Does it mean that she is less free to make a decision?

What ethical theories justify the decisions you have been making? Have you respected Ed's rights? Marta's rights? Have you done your duty as a physician? Have you overdone it? Have you done what is best for Ed? For Marta? For society as a whole?

Carefully consider these issues before you make a decision. If you decide not to remove the feeding tube, continue reading the following section. If you decide to remove the tube, turn to "Discussion."

You Just Could Not Stop the Feeding

You have decided to maintain Ed's feeding. You have placed a gastrostomy tube and sent him to a nursing home. Another several weeks have passed, and he remains stable. There is no improvement, but neither is he getting any worse.

The cost of Ed's stay in the ICU was $2,000 per day, on the regular hospital floor, $700. In the nursing home it is $300 per day. Insurance covers most of this, but Marta must pay 20 percent. Soon, however, Ed will reach the limits of his policy and the whole burden will be on Marta. She will need to spend down their assets, essentially by selling Ed's business—the money they were counting on for retirement—until Ed can qualify for Medicaid, the welfare program. Although she cannot be forced to sell their house, she will have to spend almost all their savings. Only after these resources are gone will the state take over the nursing home bills.

Can you continue to face Marta? How will you help her to bear the psychological strain of seeing Ed in a hopeless medical condition, totally dependent on the type of care he hated? Will you help her with the financial burdens involved in Ed's care?

Think of what you would say to Marta to explain why you have persisted in keeping Ed on the tube feeding. Specify the moral theory on which you based your decision. Would disconnecting Ed violate his right to life? Would it be killing him? Is feeding Ed required by your duty as a physician? Is it a benefit to him or to society?

Is there anything you will leave out of the explanation? Are you going to discuss the legal ramifications of not feeding Ed? Are you going to discuss the hospital's or your own financial interests in the case? How do your answers to these questions relate to the moral theory you are using?

Could there be a change in Ed's situation that would lead you to discontinue feeding him? Are you committed to keeping patients like Ed going no matter what else might happen, such as a heart attack? Would you consider increasing the level of therapy in that situation? How, for example, will you treat the pneumonias he will eventually develop? Will you use whatever antibiotics it will take? Do you think that it is wrong to discontinue a course of therapy once it is begun but acceptable not to begin new therapies? Use your moral theory to develop and justify this distinction. After you have thought through your explanation, continue reading the following discussion.

Discussion

You have just gone through a common scenario for many patients with strokes, severe head injuries, cardiac arrests, or even surgical misadventures. Estimates put the number of patients in a permanent vegetative state between 10,000 and 25,000.

If at any later time you decide to discontinue his feeding line, it would have been better had you done it sooner. Then you would have avoided the lengthy, useless care, the suffering of the family and, most of all, you would have followed Ed Martinez's fervent wishes. But in the operating room there was no way to know whether he would recover. Without such knowledge, not resuscitating him would not be a wise decision. Only the subsequent hours, days, or weeks would reveal the severity of the brain damage and the degree of Ed's recovery.

If Ed had awakened, the decision to keep him on the respirator would have been best. And had Ed died, had he met all the standard criteria for brain death, there would have been no moral problem. But keeping him on a respirator entails the risk that he will remain neither brain dead nor alert. The longer you maintain care, the greater the chance that he will survive in some limbo state. The demands of good emergency decision-making militate against insuring the best outcome for Ed Martinez.

Euthanasia could provide an alternative way of facing these problems in which it is possible to avoid the Hobson's choice between risking the loss of a salvageable patient and risking the survival of a patient in a persistent vegetative state. Better decisions could be made if there were more knowledge of the patient's condition and less of the pressure of an emergency. Consider the following revision of the beginning of this case.

An Alternative Approach

You leave the operating room for a discussion with Marta. Taking her from the waiting room to a conference room, you explain the anesthetic mishap and tell her that you do not know what the consequences will be. You explain that the best course of action is to provide maximum care for Ed: put him on a respirator, get an EEG, and see what happens over the next few days.

"Marta," you continue, "I think the chances of Ed's making a full recovery are small, but we should give him every chance. Despite everything we do, he may not make it. But if he survives and is severely impaired, I can assure you that he will not suffer either pain or the indignities of a severely damaged life. He does not want to live that way. And he would not want to put you through the agony of his lingering in a chronic vegetative state.

"His wish to avoid this can be accomplished swiftly and painlessly by injection once it becomes obvious that he will not regain consciousness. The hospital has a Euthanasia Committee that understands these situations. If we get to that point, the committee will review the case to insure that the family and the physicians are acting as the patient would have wanted. If we see clearly that Ed is going to be severely impaired, we can ask the committee to go over the case carefully and talk with us, affording legal protection to all concerned.

"The existence of the committee makes the present decision easy. We can go all out for Ed, giving him the best chance for a good recovery. Yet we also know that we have an escape if things do not go as we hope.

"Three or four days from now, or whenever the situation is clarified, and if things aren't going well, we'll call in the Euthanasia Committee. After consulting with them, we could turn off the respirator. If Ed breathes at this point, we could give him an injection of potassium that would stop his heart and allow him to die swiftly and painlessly.

"We won't be forced to stand by helplessly, waiting for Ed to get a pneumonia that we won't treat. Ed and everyone else will be spared the agony of a lingering, perhaps painful, death. With an injection, he can have a good death—euthanasia. That's what the term means."

*   *   *

There are no euthanasia committees; the scenario presented here is impossible under current law anywhere. No matter what your ultimate position, consider the pragmatic advantages and disadvantages of any such proposal. It would offer patients in Ed Martinez's position the most vigorous possible therapy. What would be the effect of such legislation on patients or families who would reject a euthanasia option? What safeguards would be required for the operation of such a committee? Should anyone involved be able to reject euthanasia: patient, physician, family? What should the committee do when a family is divided? How would one insure that such committees did not take advantage of the weak, the handicapped, and the defenseless? Should the committees use an adversarial system to prevent abuses?

Euthanasia—a good death—is one of the major ethical issues in American and European society. We increasingly debate whether to embark on a techno-logical intervention with medicine or machines. We vigorously debate deci-sions about discontinuing those interventions when they are shown in individ-ual cases not to be effective in "curing" the problem but only effective in preserving life. We must also consider how to allow individuals who do not require "heroic" or "extraordinary" medical intervention to die with dignity. Should they be allowed to commit suicide? Should physicians or others be able to help them die?

If you wish to support euthanasia, to what moral theory are you appealing? Do you argue that people have the right to control their own lives, and that euthanasia in these cases is like suicide—simply another instance of the right of self-determination? Would euthanasia enhance the well-being of either the individual or society? Would a euthanasia policy carry out the duty of society to respect individuals and their independence?

If you are opposed to euthanasia, what are the moral grounds of your oppo-sition? Does it violate someone's right to life, even if the person renounces that right? Does it violate the respect owed to a person? Does it violate our integrity to kill other people, no matter what the people killed might have thought? Would a policy of euthanasia inevitably lead to abusive social practices?

Finally, compare your response in this case to the response you made in Chapter 2, "Jill." What are the morally significant differences between these two cases? Do these differences cause you to come to different decisions in the two cases?

PART
II

ADULTHOOD

chapter

4

* * * * *

Leon

"It's sad to be talking to myself like this, but when there's no one else. . . .

"With the kids grown up and gone, it was only the two of us, for the first time in almost 30 years—just the two of us—no more allowances, no more tuition, no more responsibilities. We were free, not only financially free but emotionally free to do some of the things we had always planned to do or dreamed about. Now we could take that camera safari to Kenya, the trip to the Galapagos to see the tortoises. We could take the cruise in the Caribbean we had planned but had to cancel when Jody came down with the measles. It isn't fair to have Leon's health go bad when things looked so promising, when we finally had the money to live well. Now I feel all alone, faced with all these decisions. Leon's always been a fighter, and I think he'll win this one too.

"Morty—Dr. Morton—had looked after us for the past 12 years, ever since Leon found that lump in his groin. It turned out to be a lymphoma. At that time it was Morty who had found us the surgeon and then arranged for the radiotherapy. He was the one who would translate what those other doctors really meant when they said, 'There's a possibility that . . .' He would point out how that was different from when they said, 'There's a good possibility that . . .' He would patiently explain what a 5 percent chance meant, how to understand 'a 20 percent chance,' or 'a 30 percent risk of' when I only had one husband. Morty had translated all of that doctor-talk into understandable language and had helped us with the many decisions. Now that I think back on it, it was so much easier then. Everything worked out so well. Morty really made the decisions, and all I had to do was agree.

"He continued to be our friend, not just our physician. Not close friends, but we were friends—until this happened. Where was he when I really needed him? Off in some foreign country, enjoying himself. He may not even know what has happened. But it's hard to keep your faith in doctors after all we've been through in the past six months.

"Leon wasn't doing well this past summer and had some headaches. He went to Dr. Morton's office in August, and Morty said that he was probably just worn down. 'Maybe you should get away,' he said. Perhaps the strain was causing migraine headaches. 'If the headaches aren't better after Labor Day when I get back,' he said, 'I'll run some tests.'

"Leon took a few days off, but the headaches didn't seem to get better. Then there were several days when he didn't seem himself. I had a call from his law partner asking if things were okay at home. I didn't know what he meant. He said that Leon was talking strangely at times, and for the past few days, he said, Leon was very forgetful. When I asked, Leon said it was the migraines. But he began to stumble, and then he hit his head. We called Morton's office and they sent us for a brain scan. Can you imagine, the office sent us for a brain scan without ever seeing us, without a doctor's even examining Leon! It wouldn't have happened if Dr. Morton had been in town.

"It was the look on that radiologist's face that first told us there was trouble. He asked us the name of our physician and we didn't know what name to give him. Dr. Morton was still out of town. The next day, one of our friends gave us the name of a doctor he knew, and through him we got Dr. Neville, who became our neurosurgeon. You have really hit rock bottom when a family has their own neurosurgeon. Dr. Neville seemed wonderful; he really took charge of the situation. He said we really didn't have a choice. He had already put the biopsy on the schedule for the morning.

"'A biopsy is a small procedure,' I remember him saying. 'After putting Leon to sleep, we make a small hole in the skull and take a tiny piece of tissue so that we can examine it under the microscope. That way we'll be able to determine what's causing the problem and how best to treat it.'

"He made it all sound so simple. We were grateful to be in such competent hands. It's funny how clearly that conversation has stayed in my mind."

* * *

Contemporary medical ethics requires that patients or their representatives be fully informed before embarking on any therapy, that they give their informed consent.

As a patient, how much information do you want? Do you want all the information about all the risks of the biopsy and their consequences? Do you really want to know all the risks and the consequences of not doing the surgery and its alternatives? Do you really want to be the one deciding what should be done on the basis of all that information? Do you want physicians to give you the facts, or do you want their opinions as well?

As a physician, how would you assess what patients want regarding decision-making? Should you provide them with only the information that you believe helpful and appropriate? Should you give them all the relevant information, but then advise them plainly on what you think is the best course?

What are the boundaries of "relevant," and who should determine those boundaries? How would you handle the under-informed? The over-informed?

As an ethicist, would you say that informed consent is a minimal requirement, a realistic goal, or an unrealistic ideal?

Put yourself in Leon's wife's position and decide what you want done. Would you go along with Dr. Neville's recommendation, or do you and Leon want to decide for yourselves?

- If you feel that you are adequately informed and grateful that Dr. Neville has made the decision so much easier, go home and get a good night's sleep. Then go to "Scenario 1" and read on.
- If you are overwhelmed by what has happened, and want more time to gather information, then ask Dr. Neville if you can sleep on the decision overnight and discuss it with your children in the morning. Then go to "Scenario 2" and read on.
- If you prefer to get another opinion, tell Dr. Neville that you want a second opinion and either ask him for the names of other good neurosurgeons, or call some of your friends and see who they would recommend. Then go to "Scenario 3" and read on.

There are, of course, other possibilities, but let's limit our choices to these three.

Scenario 1

"It's hard to remember back to that night, but I think that I said, 'Thank you, Dr. Neville. Yes.' And 'Tomorrow?' and 'What time?' and 'I'll see you in the morning.' Now that I think about it, perhaps I was too grateful, too passive. If I hadn't been so overwhelmed, so willing to let Dr. Neville make the decisions, perhaps things would have turned out differently."

Now turn to "Following the Biopsy," and read on.

Scenario 2

"Dr. Neville, It has been such a hard day. I'm so tired, and Leon is falling asleep. Do we have to make a decision tonight? Our children will be here in the morning and we could talk it over. Is it an emergency? Or can it wait a bit?"

"Well, you never know with these things," Dr. Neville responded. "We don't know how long it's been there. We know Leon's gotten worse these past several weeks, even over the past several days. I'd advise doing the biopsy tomorrow so that we can begin the treatment as soon as possible. But if you insist, we can postpone it for a few days. I'll reschedule the biopsy for Monday morning; that will give you three days to consider it. In the meantime we'll start some steroids to decrease the swelling. Perhaps he'll feel a bit better too."

"Next morning Leon was eating breakfast when I arrived with the morning paper. He looked better than he had in weeks. 'I don't know what they gave me last night,' he said quite cheerfully, 'The whole day is a blur, but I feel great this morning. Neville seemed like a nice guy, but I think I fell asleep while he was talking. What did he say, and when can I get out of here?'

"Andy and Paula both arrived about an hour later and were very upset that I hadn't called them sooner. I explained to them about the headaches and the stumbling, and then about the brain scan. I told them that Dr. Neville had wanted to do a biopsy this morning, but that I had wanted to discuss it with them before making a decision.

"Andy wanted to know about the risks of the biopsy. What could it show us that would change the way we were managing the problem? Did Dr. Neville think that it was cancer? If so, would it require another operation? What were the chances of a cure? What were the other possibilities? If steroids could make dad so much better, why did we need to rush?

"When he came by later that morning, Dr. Neville responded patiently to these questions. He said that the biopsy was a small, routine procedure, something that he did several times a week. That there was always a risk to anesthesia, but the risks of the biopsy itself were very small. He emphasized that the biopsy was the only way to determine what type of cancer this was, and was absolutely necessary before they could decide about further surgery, radiation, or chemotherapy. The steroids had relieved the brain swelling but had not cured the problem.

"Several of our physician friends heard of Leon's admission and stopped by. I don't know if they were a help or not. Each meant well. Each knew a little bit about Leon's problems. Every one of them knew another physician who was up on the latest treatment for . . . for what? We still didn't even know what Leon had. After talking to each one I had lots more information, but I didn't feel better informed.

"We were deciding the answer to a very simple question requiring a yes or no answer. Should we let Dr. Neville do the biopsy—or not?"

* * *

If you now feel sufficiently informed and decide to proceed with the biopsy, turn to "Following the Biopsy," and read on.

If you decide to seek a second opinion, read "Scenario 3."

Scenario 3

Dr. G. Hugo Wallach was impeccably dressed as befits the senior neuro-surgeon in town. In his early 60s, with silver gray hair, Dr. Wallach had been the chief of neurosurgery until his retirement several years ago. An avid golfer and a middling tennis player, he could be found most afternoons at the country club, either out on the course or in the club room playing bridge. It was after the bridge game that he had been cajoled into coming down to the hospital to see Leon and render a second opinion.

"I'm retired, you realize, and I no longer operate, but for a friend of a golfing partner, I sometimes bend my self-imposed rules about practicing medicine after age 60."

He listened thoughtfully to the history and then carefully studied the MRI scan. "Hmm," he mumbled. "He plans to biopsy that spot. I wouldn't do that if I were the surgeon. I don't have that much courage. But these younger guys, they use the MRIs like road maps and just charge ahead. With as few problems as Leon has, I'd just sit tight for a few days and see how the steroids work. Back in the old days, before we had these MRIs, we would have given Leon some aspirin and seen him back in a few days. I might repeat the scan next week to see if anything's changed. If it really is a tumor, another week is not going to make much difference. Given its location it would be impossible to get it all out. So you'll end up with chemotherapy and radiation anyway, whatever the biopsy shows, and the therapy will give him a few extra months. Most tumors in a location like that aren't curable, but I'm not even sure it is a tumor. I once had a patient with a lesion like that and it just disappeared. It must have been some type of inflammation. I think there is not much to be lost by waiting and repeating the scan next week."

* * *

Now that you have your second opinion, what will you do? Which of these surgeons is giving the best advice? How do you know?

Was it ethical for Dr. Neville to push for early surgery? Had he really informed you and let you weigh the risks? Is Dr. Wallach just practicing old-fashioned medicine and ignoring the advances that MRI scans have brought to the early detection of lesions?

If you feel that you were adequately informed after discussing the risks and benefits with Dr. Neville, how do you reconcile that with the very different information you were given by Dr. Wallach? If you received new information, then you couldn't have been fully informed previously. Or perhaps Wallach is giving you misinformation? How do you test the quality of the information you have received? What do you do now? Get a third opinion and vote?

If you've decided to follow Dr. Neville's advice and proceed with the biopsy read "Following the Biopsy." If you decide to follow Dr. Wallach's advice turn to "Wallach's Outcome."

Following the Biopsy

"The biopsy went smoothly. Dr. Neville came out afterwards and told us everything had gone well. He said that the frozen sections looked like some form of a lymphoma, but they couldn't be sure. The permanent sections should be ready next week; then the pathologist could tell better. It might even be a recurrence of that old problem in his groin. In the meantime he would do tests to look for where it might have come from. Chest x-ray, bone scans, radioactive something-or-others, enemas, swallows. I don't even remember half of them.

"All I remember was that Leon didn't wake up. Leon did not wake up! Nobody told me that could happen. The first afternoon they said that it was still the effect of the anesthetic and that he should be fine that evening. That evening they took him back for another brain scan to be sure there wasn't bleeding or anything—there wasn't. He'll be awake by morning, they assured me. I spent the night in the waiting room outside of the intensive care unit and every hour, or every ten minutes—I don't even know—I'd ask and they would say, 'He's resting quietly.'

"When Neville came by early the next morning, he told me that Leon was in a coma. *Coma!* I was on the verge of hysteria. I didn't have anyone to turn to help me. 'Coma,' Dr. Neville said, 'is just like sleeping . . .'—except you don't wake up. I've learned a lot of medicine since that day. Neville went on to explain that the 'lesion,' that's what they call the 'bad cells,' was right next to the brain stem, the area that controls alertness, breathing, and all that important stuff. He said that perhaps there was just some swelling due to the biopsy and that Leon should wake up in a few days when the swelling went down. In the meantime we would wait for the results of the biopsy. He would perform those other tests and consult with the tumor specialist to decide whether to start radiotherapy or chemotherapy.

"The following Tuesday Dr. Neville asked us to meet him at five in the evening for a conference. The kids were there, and my brother Joe had come in. Neville brought a young doctor who was a medical oncologist, a doctor who specializes in the treatment of tumors with chemicals instead of radiation. She introduced herself and in her quiet, gentle manner explained that the tumor appeared to be a lymphoma. She said that lymphomas rarely start in the brain, they usually spread from somewhere else in the body, but so far all of the other tests had been negative. They couldn't find where the tumor had started, but the good news was that with lymphomas it probably didn't matter. If we used a radiotherapy in combination with various chemotherapies—she called it a 'protocol' and it had a number—we had a good chance of getting the primary tumor as well as treating these various lesions in the brain.

"Andy asked about his chances, and she seemed optimistic. I guess we weren't sufficiently sophisticated to ask her what she was optimistic about or what she meant when she said that she was optimistic. Now I know to ask doctors what they mean when they use these sorts of words because words seem to mean very different things when they are used by the medical profession. I've learned to make the doctors be very specific. As I look back on it now, even when Dr. Neville said that he still thought Leon would wake up, I was assuming that the old Leon would still be there and that one morning when I came in, he would smile and say, 'Good Morning!' I came in every morning, but Leon was still 'asleep.'

"They started the chemotherapy and the radiotherapy, but Leon slept through it all. I stayed awake for both of us. After the third week a few friends began to ask me how long they expected before the treatment would begin to work. Were the doctors still hopeful? Had we ever discussed stopping the treatments? I wanted to shout: *No,* we aren't going to quit! not while there was a chance of the treatment working. Not while there was a chance that Leon would wake up. Leon and I hadn't even had a chance to say good-bye. It had all been so sudden, just a biopsy—then this. Dr. Neville was still optimistic—I think. He would stop by every two or three days, now that Leon had left the intensive care unit and moved to the Cancer Center. Our very nice medical oncologist left on vacation, and her assistant, I can't remember his name, came in her place every day but he said that he was 'just covering.' Any major decisions would have to wait for her return.

"Time and life seemed to drag on. The kids had gone back to their work, but they called almost every day. There wasn't much to say. Our friends were terrific, but sitting around Leon's room didn't give me much to talk about. We seemed to avoid talking about the only thing that was really important to me. What was there to say? Leon was still asleep. It looked as if the 'lesion' in the brain was shrinking. Or at least wasn't getting any larger which, I was told, must mean that the treatment was working. It was only a matter of time. Time for what?

"I found myself silently asking Leon to show me that he was still there. Just some little sign. An eye blink, a smile, a groan, anything at all—anything except that unwavering stare. Please! No one had ever warned me that this could happen, like suspended animation. I didn't know what to hope for any more. Anything but this. . . . If we could just have said good-bye, then I could rest more easily.

"During the week before Thanksgiving, I was making out the shopping list for dinner with the family. Andy would be here, and Paula with her girls. We would try to make it as festive as possible under the circumstances. At first I thought there was some response as I described the dinner to Leon. The next day I was almost certain. On the day before Thanksgiving he definitely looked at me when I spoke. It had been almost ten weeks. I think that almost everyone had given up, everyone but me. I told you Leon was a fighter! Thanksgiving turned out to be festive after all. The girls climbed all over Leon's bed and he seemed to enjoy it. Every day after that things continued to improve. By the first of December he could carry on a conversation. Well, it was a bit one-sided, but he clearly seemed to understand what people were saying. He would smile and even answer questions although it was often difficult to understand what he was trying to say. He'd become very frustrated when I didn't understand. The therapy had finished, and now we could make plans to go home.

"The social worker helped put us in touch with the home health care group. We arranged for a hospital bed in the living room, a wheelchair, two shifts of nursing help, and a list of what seemed like a thousand other things. But at least, at last, Leon would be back home.

"Eventually we canceled our trip to the Galapagos. Clearly, Leon could not go, and anyway we could no longer afford it. Despite Medicare, the home nursing care rapidly ate up our savings and we didn't know how long this would go on. I enjoyed having Leon home to talk to and to help care for, even though the conversations remained one-sided. We went for our walks, Leon in his chair. The kids all came for his birthday in July, and he seemed to enjoy having them around. But it was hard to tell for sure. It certainly wasn't what we had planned.

"On balance life had returned to a reasonable equilibrium, but at times I couldn't help but wonder what would have happened if I had made a different decision that first night. Was I well informed when I decided about the biopsy? I don't know. Even now, I don't know now if I wanted to be informed—or wanted to be more informed. Did I really want to know that the risk of one outcome was 12 percent and that the chances of something else happening were 17 percent? I remember being totally overwhelmed that night and thinking that I could never learn enough to make the right decision. Even now, having been through it, I'm not sure I know what was the right decision for Leon. Of course, we wanted to give Leon every chance. I think that the doctor did exactly what I wanted, but, if he hadn't been so definite about the need for a biopsy, if we had gotten a second opinion, maybe things would have turned out differently.

Dr. Wallach's Outcome

"After Dr. Wallach's more optimistic opinion, and with Leon looking so well after the steroids, we thought that we would wait to see what that next week would bring. Over the next few days Leon's strength continued to improve and he went home. No more headaches, no more stumbling, no problems with his memory. Two weeks later we went back for another scan and, much to everyone's amazement, it was much improved. Dr. Neville said it was unbelievable; he could barely see a trace where the lesion had been. 'I've hardly ever seen anything like it,' he said. 'It must not have been a tumor, or it must have been very steroid-sensitive.'

As Dr. Wallach had said, inflammation occasionally simulates tumors and disappears. As I write this, we are sitting on the deck of the cruise ship having spent the morning watching the tortoises.

*   *   *

Informed Consent

No one should ever be subjected to surgery or any medical treatment without their informed consent. Kant's principle of respect for persons demands that we treat others as responsible human beings who can make significant decisions about their own lives. Utilitarian principles suggest that, in the long run, well-informed patients are happier. In contemporary research ethics, a participant must be fully informed about the potential risks and benefits of experimental treatment and sign a form which has been preapproved by a supervising committee.

Few principles in medicine are as widely accepted as that of informed consent, but there is no accepted moral standard of how informed the patient must be. There is a legal standard that a patient should be as informed as a "reasonable person" would want to be. But this is not practically clear since it depends on how a judge or jury interprets the idea of the "reasonable person," which they do in various ways. In response to surveys, patients routinely say they want to be more fully informed. But widespread clinical experience indicates that patients' desire for and ability to absorb more information is limited. This raises moral questions: when is the patient treated with the respect every human being deserves, and when are physicians stepping over the line into paternalism or coercion?

Every treatment or procedure has side effects. Some occur frequently and are usually not serious. Some are rare but very serious—death from an operation, hepatitis from a medication. Coma after biopsy, like Leon's, is rare and unexpected. Should Dr. Neville have warned Leon's family of this remote possibility? If so, he would have had to inform her of myriad other rare and unanticipated events as well and she, like most of us, would have been overwhelmed.

In Scenario 1, Dr. Neville simplified the risks and the benefits to fit a short time frame and essentially assumed responsibility for guiding the decision toward what he believed needed to be done. Was this behavior wrong? Was it objectionably paternalistic or was it following the principle of beneficence that requires physicians to act for the benefit of their patients?

In Scenario 2 the perceived pressure of time has been removed since Leon is better on the steroids. Leon's children are there to support their mother and to ask additional questions. At the end of this discussion, is everyone adequately informed? Is the outcome of the biopsy different?

According to the Nuremberg Code, informed consent requires that choices not involve duress, excessive pressure, or coercion. In Scenario 1, did Dr. Neville exert excessive pressure to have the biopsy done? Was their consent truly voluntary? Did removing the pressure of time in Scenario 2 and answering all of the questions allow a more voluntary consent?

Following is one more attempt to produce an informed decision.

Scenario 4

Dr. Neville sits down in Leon's room, leans forward, and says: "We have a very serious problem here. There is a lesion in Leon's brain which is very close to the brain stem, the vital center of brain function. I don't know what it is. I think that it is a tumor, and it may be related to the tumors Leon had in the past. I hope so, because lymphomas are very sensitive to radiation and to chemotherapy. If it is a lymphoma, we have a good chance of giving Leon many more good years. If it is some other type of malignancy, things would not look so good, since it is so close to the brain stem that I doubt that I could take it all out. In either case, however, we need to do the biopsy, since it is the only way of knowing the tumor type, and the oncologist will not give either radiation or chemotherapy without knowing the tumor type. You have to understand that even the biopsy is risky. I do them routinely, but in this location—in addition to the routine risks of anesthesia which include brain damage and even death—there are additional risks because of the tumor's location. These include bleeding into the brain which would damage the brain stem. From such an injury, Leon might die or never wake up. He might be in a coma for a short or a very long time if things go badly. And then there is always the risk of infection. If you add all of these things together, I would give him at least a 90 to 95 percent chance of doing well. There's a 2 to 3 percent chance of having some minor complication, and a 1 to 2 percent chance of something seriously bad happening. Think it over with your children, and let me know tomorrow. It looks as if we have some time. Do you have any more questions?"

Dr. Neville stands, shake hands with everyone and starts to leave. He then pops back in and says, "Just remember, if we don't do the biopsy, we won't know the type of tumor, and we won't be able to give the chemotherapy."

*   *   *

Is this "fully informed consent"? Has Dr. Neville fulfilled his duty to respect the autonomy of Leon and his family? Will Leon's wife be happier when Leon doesn't wake up?

chapter

5

* * * * *

Ms. Williams

Ethics is more than confronting extraordinary moral dilemmas and making difficult decisions; it also concerns the process by which everyday decisions are made (see Chapter 19). The ethical practice of medicine includes the art of developing an effective relationship between patients and physicians, a relationship in which both are comfortable. The scenarios in this chapter, as in Chapter 11, raise issues that are not usually addressed by principle-based ethics, but are nevertheless genuine moral concerns.

Many of the current moral judgments made about physicians and medical care rest on differences of expectation between patients and physicians. Autonomy has become the watchword in medicine, and especially in medical ethics. Some people put a high priority on expertise, others on compassion, while paternalism and benevolence have become dirty words for many who see these qualities as enemies of autonomous decision-making.

What sort of a physician would you choose for yourself and your family? From the list that follows, pick the three most prominent qualities you want when choosing your physician.

Compassionate	Competent	Caring
Honest	Paternalistic	Maternal
Expert	Beneficent	Objective

Here are some brief definitions of these terms:

Beneficent: doing good, expressing active kindness
Caring: acting from interest or concern for others
Compassion: participation in another's suffering; sympathy
Competent: having the requisite skill, properly qualified
Expert: one with the status of an authority by reason of special training or knowledge
Honest: truthful, marked by uprightness and probity

Maternal: having the instincts of a mother
Objective: expressing facts without distortion by personal feelings or bias
Paternalistic: regulating the conduct or lives of others for their benefit

The relationship between these qualities and the realities of today's family life and medical practice is very complex. But the stereotypes associated with some terms pose problems for physicians and medical practice. The term *paternalism* conjures up the image of stern, Victorian fatherhood, for example the father in Mary Poppins. Meanwhile Mary Poppins herself, the children's nanny, is an ideal of warm and tender maternal love.

Patients often want physicians to provide comfort and the security of expertise. They go to a physician expecting a gentle but guiding hand. Prior generations of physicians prided themselves on knowing and acting in their patients' best interest. Physicians are now asking patients to provide the guidance that many patients were accustomed to expect from the medical profession. At the very least, the difference in expectation can produce severe communication problems.

How should physicians relate to those who come to them for care? Should they treat them as "patients," as "clients," or as "health care consumers." Should the setting in which physicians work—city emergency room, rural clinic, private pediatric office—structure this interaction? Given the diversity of American life and medical culture, is there a coherent ideal of the good physician? Without such an ideal, how is it possible for physicians in training to get a clear sense of what is expected of them?

The purpose of this discussion is to stimulate your thinking about the ethics and styles of medicine. Whether you are a physician, a medical or pre-med student, a nurse or student nurse, or simply a resident of this country who will someday need medical attention, your expectations for the care you give or receive are critical. What do you want from medicine, and what does it want from you?

*   *   *

Mary Williams, 42, has found a small lump in her breast. She has moved to the area only recently, so she turns to the yellow pages to find a gynecologist. The following scenarios depict three different physicians and their responses when facing the same clinical situation.

Dr. Ames

"Mary, there is a small shadow on the mammogram, and I think I can feel the tiny lump you discovered. You were very good to pick it up. The mammogram doesn't tell us what it is, but I don't think it's anything to worry about. Just to be safe, I think that we should get a biopsy of the tissue, then we can talk about what we've found and the best way to proceed. Is that okay with you?

"I'll schedule the biopsy as soon as possible so you won't be worrying. Perhaps we can do it next week. Bring someone with you to drive you home. The office will call you with the time, and you can talk to the nurse who will give you a lot of the details about what to expect."

* * *

In this brief presentation by Dr. Ames, do you detect caring, compassion, and concern in the physician? Are you on a first-name basis with your physician? Should he be on a first-name basis with you? Was Dr. Ames being paternalistic? Condescending? If he thinks that the lump has a small chance of being a cancer, was he being protective and paternalistic in his approach when he avoided giving Mary potentially frightening information? Is this the correct way to allow her to be fully informed? Do you think he was honest with Mary? Does honesty require him to provide all the statistical information based on age, location, and size of the lump? If he really thinks it may be cancer, should he be telling her, or do you think it may be kinder to defer the possible bad news until he knows for sure. If he thinks it is unlikely to be a cancer, what do you think he should be telling her?

* * *

Dr. Baker

"Ms. Williams have a seat over there, on the other side of my desk," says Dr. Baker as he settles into his deeply cushioned executive chair.

"There is a shadow on your mammogram, Ms. Williams. Your x-ray is the fourth one from the left on the wall over there. We do a lot of mammograms in this office. I can show it to you, if you like, but frankly it takes a lot of training and experience to learn how to read a mammogram. Of course, an x-ray can't tell for sure whether what I'm seeing is cancerous. It could be just a cyst. A biopsy is required for a definitive diagnosis, but cancer is definitely a possibility. I'm sure you are quite nervous, most women are at this stage, so we'll do that biopsy as soon as possible.

"If the biopsy does show cancer, then there will be several different ways to handle it. I like my patients to be fully informed as they make their decisions. We participate in some of the country's most advanced cancer research protocols, and informed consent is a prerequisite for participation. We have a handout on how to get psychologically ready for the biopsy. I'd like you to be sure to read that one; you'll find it helpful.

"You also need to know that, if the biopsy is positive, we'll want to move quickly. That's another reason I'm giving you all these details now. Again, the nurse will give you some handouts with the latest information about the various alternatives if this should be cancer. After you've read them, you may call the office with questions, and my team will answer them. This way you can think about the various options ahead of time.

"Depending on the biopsy, it may be that removing a part of the breast is an option, and some surgeons are just removing the lump. When we know more about the cancer, its receptor sites and immunologic characteristics, we can talk and decide what is best for you. Another option is a radical mastectomy with removal of the lymph nodes on the chest wall and under your arm. That is probably the most complete surgery we can do, but even that does not assure a cure. We will be able to tell more when we study the lymph nodes pathologically.

"It is important for you to understand the risks and the outcomes of each of these possibilities, and there are others, including some of the ongoing research protocols. The many studies which have been completed each have different rates of short- and long-term survival as well as different side effects.

"My nurse will give you the literature about these alternatives. See you on Tuesday at 7:30 A.M., and remember to follow all the instructions on the handout.

"Doris, can you give Ms. Williams our biopsy and breast cancer packets, and bring my next patient back. Thanks."

* * *

This brief excerpt of Dr. Baker's presentation has a very different tone than Dr. Ames's. The future, with the various surgical alternatives, is mentioned, and literature with more information is provided. Mary could ask questions of the nurse if she felt she needed more information. Would you prefer this approach? We don't know Dr. Baker's thoughts about the chance that this small lump is malignant. If he thinks the chance is small, has his detailed approach to laying out the future helped Mrs. Williams to be a more informed participant in the decisions which may or may not lie ahead?

Is his approach paternalistic? Should physicians force patients to think about the possible long-term consequences of the biopsy, even at the cost of the short-term anxiety? Was this a compassionate discussion? What are Dr. Baker's good qualities? What qualities does he lack? Which qualities does Mary's life depend on, his good qualities or his weaknesses?

Was honesty one of the attributes that you most wanted in your physician? What is honesty in the face of uncertainty?

* * *

Dr. Charles

"Mary, there is no way to tell for sure, but I'm thinking that this is more than likely just a cyst, nothing to worry about," says Dr. Charles, taking

Mary's hand gently. The mammogram doesn't show much, and I think that the most conservative approach is to just watch it. I suppose that it could be a cancer, but I really don't think so. If you find it getting bigger, come back. We can see you in a month, and if nothing changes repeat the mammogram in three months. Cysts are common at your age. Some doctors jump in and do biopsies and that sort of thing, but I think the chance of its being cancer are small and we can wait a bit—if that's all right with you. Talk it over with your husband and with some of your friends, and let me know. Any questions?"

*   *   *

What does Dr. Charles really think? Is she playing the odds that this is just a cyst, doing so at the risk of Mary's life? Is her tone and demeanor more maternal, warmer and more caring? Does it show more compassion? Is there more virtue in being maternal than paternal? Has she been irresponsible by going on her instincts rather than being certain that this isn't a cancer? Was she just trying to protect Mary? Does the fact that she is a woman enter into her presentation?

*   *   *

Some patients want a lot of medical information; others want psychological assurance. Some want both, others neither. Since patients want different types and levels of help, how are physicians to know what to tell which patient? Which discussion and which physician would you prefer? Are you satisfied with any of the discussions?

Compare these three physicians by giving each a score on the following traits (make 1 the highest score and 4 the lowest)

	Dr. A.	Dr. B.	Dr. C.
Honesty			
Compassion			
Caring			
Competence			
Paternalism			
Maternalism			
Beneficence			
Expertise			
Objectivity			

Think about honesty. Which one of these physicians was most honest? Does honesty require telling the whole truth? At this stage in the evaluation, what is the whole truth? If we assume that each physician believed that the shadow on the mammogram had the same chance of being cancer, is each physician justified in giving the information from his or her own perspective only? Would it confuse patients to hear multiple possibilities or would they be reassured that all their options were discussed?

Assume that the x-ray suggested a harmless cyst, and reconsider the presentations. Now which presentation do you prefer? Which was the most honest? Which the most compassionate?

Conclusion

We think it is important that medical ethics not be confined to the narrow range of issues that can be discussed in clear terms of moral principles. The virtue tradition has recently reemerged in medical ethics (see Chapter 18), renewing interest in a number of issues. In their book *The Virtues in Medical Practice*, Edmund Pellegrino and David Thomasma show how this tradition, neglected in the last 25 years of emphasis on principle-based ethics, has important things to say about medical practice. We expect virtue ethics to play an increasingly important role in answering questions of what qualities patients should look for in physicians, and vice versa.

Given the diversity of American life and medical culture, is there a coherent ideal of the good physician? Without such an ideal, how can patients know what to expect from their doctors? Perhaps more important for some readers of this book, how is it possible for physicians or nurses to get a clear sense of what is expected of them?

chapter

6

* * * * *

Wanda

Mary and I were married during the first year of my residency; Zack was born soon after. One hundred thousand dollars in debt, we decided that we couldn't afford my taking any specialty training. We had to have an income. As soon as I finished three years in general internal medicine, I came to Whiteford.

Plain and simple, Whiteford needed a doctor and I needed a job to pay off my debts. The West Whiteford Outreach Clinic is part of a federally funded project to meet the needs of the underserved. In return for working with this population, the government forgives a portion of medical school loans, and the clinic's doctor receives a reasonable salary. It's not a bad living. The doctor who had just left spent three years here, and paid off enough debt to afford to open her own practice in a more affluent place downstate. That is how my new job opened up.

From its main street, Whiteford looks like a New England town with charming shops and white clapboard houses. The riverfront tells a different story; two decades ago the first of the mills moved out and many people followed. Those who stayed were either rich enough that they didn't have to move or so poor that they couldn't. The West Whiteford Outreach Clinic was part of the town's attempt to serve those who couldn't move. The clinic has one physician—me—and some night and weekend coverage by other doctors from up the hill. There are two very dedicated nurses and a secretary who has been with the clinic for 15 years. I'd been there about a week when Wanda came in.

An attractive young woman, she was sitting on the examining table with Jenny, one of the nurses, at her side and a sheriff's deputy slouched in a corner chair.

"Why are you here, Wanda?" I asked.

After I got no response to several questions, the deputy spoke up, "She says she's got headaches, and the sheriff wants you to check her out."

"Do you have headaches, Wanda?"

"No."

"Are you sure?"

"No!"

"Then why are you screaming every morning?" said the deputy, "and driving all the other prisoners nuts? You keep yelling that your head is killing you. There's got to be something wrong."

"Why is she in jail?" I asked.

"She's been in jail for about a week for biting a worker at the group home. The lady's pressing charges, says she's fed up with Wanda and all the abuse she gives everyone. Fighting, swearing, running away. The home doesn't want her back, and her mom doesn't want her either. That's why she's still in jail; no one would bail her out."

"Do you have headaches, Wanda?" I asked again in my most patient voice.

"Only when they won't let me do what I want. Then I yell back and I puke all over them."

"What do they want you to do?"

"They want me to get up and clean the cell and get dressed and everything before they give me breakfast. They shout at me and it gives me a headache, and I just yell and scream back at them so they'll take me down to the infirmary where I can lie down. The nurse is nice to me."

"I see," I mumbled as I began to write down a problem list.

Wanda _____

21 year old. Headaches in morning. Vomiting, probably stress-related . . .

As I was writing this note, I was thinking, "What is the proper approach to this problem? The headaches are probably Wanda's way of coping with the demands at the jail. They get her out of doing unpleasant things and allow her to lie down in a nicer environment. On the other hand, the first sign of a brain tumor is early-morning headaches and vomiting. A tumor is possible, but very unlikely. Should I order a brain scan? What if I miss something? Could the clinic be sued?

"Okay," I said, aloud, "problem number one is the headaches. Problem number two is what to do with Wanda so she doesn't have to stay in jail. Why are you in trouble?" I asked.

"I bit the lady," said Wanda, "and she got mad, so I runned away."

"We picked her up near Lacy's Diner," added the officer. "That's where she usually turns up."

"Why did you bite the lady?"

"She was pushing on me again. She wanted me to clean up after dinner. She said that I couldn't watch TV until the whole kitchen was clean and neat. She was making me sick. So I bit her. The doctor told me that if I bit people or slept with them they could get really sick. I wanted her to get really sick."

"Well," I turned to Jenny, "if she can't go back to the group home, aren't there other places to send her? She's 21 now, perhaps we can get her placed somewhere else. Does Whiteford have any other place that will take her?"

"Nobody else will take her because of her self-destructive behaviors, her scratching and bleeding, and her HIV; everyone is afraid of getting it. The group home was the only one that would keep her, and now they want her out. She keeps running away. Every time she feels stressed, she goes back to see her mom. When that doesn't work out, she runs again. She hitches rides on Route 93 by shacking up with the truck drivers. It's likely that she has infected half the truckers in this part of the state."

"What's going on here?" said the deputy, dropping the ancient copy of *People* magazine she had picked up from the waiting room. "You mean Wanda's got AIDS? Nobody from the home told us at the jail. The sheriff will really want to know this."

"Tell the sheriff it's HIV, not AIDS. Tell him to call me," I responded. I asked Jenny, "Hasn't anyone taught her about HIV and sex?"

"Tell the doctor, Wanda." Jenny said by way of reply.

"They said that I got the HIVs. But if I use a rubber, everything's okay. At least unless I bite somebody, or scratch them or something. And I don't do that unless they're really mean."

"Uh," I mumbled. "This is going to take a lot longer than I thought. We better spend some time sorting everything out. I don't think that there's anything to worry about with the headaches. She doesn't need any tests right now. When she screams at the jail, let her go down to the infirmary, at least until we work out her other problems. I think that the headaches and the vomiting are Wanda's very effective way of manipulating her environment. As far as the residential settings, her HIV and her transmission of it to others, we better get some help from the county's social service department. Jenny, could you contact somebody down there to see if we can set up a meeting for tomorrow morning before the clinic opens.

"Wanda, now I want you to behave better at the jail. No more of this screaming and biting. I'll try to help you. We're going to talk with some people tomorrow and see if we can't find you a nice place to live. Would you like that?"

Without waiting for an answer, I left for my office and a cup of coffee. Fortunately the next patient hadn't shown up, so I had ten minutes to myself to think and to finish my notes.

Wanda _____
21-year-old female. Headaches in morning. Vomiting, probably stress

related. Mild retardation, self-destructive behavior, biting, scratching, running away. HIV-positive. Sexually active.

Problem 1. Headaches. Wait and see how they develop. Will probably go away. Consider scan if they continue.

Problem 2. Need to find living arrangement. Protect her.

Problem 3. HIV infection. Need to protect caretakers, need to protect community. Consider "least restrictive environment." Meeting tomorrow to resolve.

* * *

It is still not clear to me how the word got out. I didn't say anything about it to anyone, but when I arrived at the clinic the next morning about 8 A.M., the parking lot was almost full, and the small conference room was overflowing. There was Roger Goudenough, vice president of the clinic's board and an attorney for the Whiteford National Bank. I had met him when I was applying for the job. Dr. Kandelbaum, the county's public health officer, was there. I'd never met him, but they said he had held the job for the last 30 years because he never made a decision. Jenny was waiting for me near the door. Outside, in a loud discussion, were Mr. Weithorson, chairman of the clinic's board, and someone else who, I later found out, was the county social worker assigned to Wanda.

Jenny whispered to me, "Look out, this place is a minefield. I didn't think word would get out or I would have warned you yesterday."

I went to the head of the table and called the group to order. As I began to introduce myself, I got my introduction to the politics of administration. Weithorson interrupted:

"Thank you, Doctor. I am glad you all could come this morning. This is a very important meeting because it may affect the future of the West Whiteford Outreach Clinic. As most of you know, and as I'm sure you are aware, Doctor, this clinic is partially funded by federal funds, but it would not be able to continue without the generous contributions of some of our leading citizens. Some of these individuals have very strong feelings about some of the issues which are going to be discussed this morning. I have come because I want to be certain that everyone here is sensitive to their concerns. Now Doctor, you may proceed."

"Thank you, Sir." I was almost on the verge of my old stammer. "I didn't expect all of you here this morning. I requested this meeting of the staff and the social workers to get a better grip on the alternatives for Wanda. Let me briefly recap the problems facing us: The group home doesn't want Wanda, our patient, back because of her behavior, and presumably because of her HIV status. Jail isn't the proper place for her either. I am concerned for her welfare. I'm also concerned about the public health implications of her sexual promiscuity. I gather it's no secret in this community that Wanda picks up truckers along the highway. We saw her yesterday because of headaches, but they don't seem to be a medical problem and—"

"Doctor," interrupted Weithorson, "we are very pleased to have you and your lovely wife in Whiteford, and I am personally delighted to see that the state's medical school continues to produce dedicated young people like you. However, this is a *medical* clinic. It has been set up to assure that, to the best of this town's ability, those who are less fortunate than ourselves do not suffer. This clinic is not a social service agency, and the social ills which have befallen our society are well beyond the capacity of our small medical facility to change. Perhaps that is the role of the county's social service agency. I do not pretend to know or to understand this generation and its behavior. What I do know is that, if this young lady is not medically ill, then she should not be the concern of this clinic and its staff. If clinic staff has so much free time to meddle in other people's business, then perhaps we do not need this amount of staff."

"If you continued to use the medical model, then I would agree with you," said the social worker. "But physical and social well-being are only different sides of the same coin. If we can't help Wanda to cope with the demands of her social environment, then she will run away again. Another trucker may become infected and no one knows how many he'll infect. Then we will all be paying the price. But our primary concern should be Wanda because she is the innocent victim of this tragedy. She is HIV-infected through no fault of her own. She has intellectual problems and behavior problems that are not her fault either. Wanda's retardation may well be the result of her parents' alcohol and drug abuse. Her behavior is largely the result of her mother's and father's physical abuse. Her HIV is also due to abuse by her father or other men in her mother's house. The group home doesn't have the personnel to provide the one-on-one care that Wanda would need to reshape her behavior. The home is not abusing her; it's merely understaffed. The state doesn't have the money to pay for the care Wanda needs. It's more expensive to keep her in jail than in the sort of home we would like, but jail comes from a different budget. More money is spent on prisoners than on the mentally handicapped, and sometimes I think that the prisoners are treated a whole lot better, especially in terms of respecting their rights."

Dr. Kandelbaum from the Public Health Department had his hand up for a while, patiently waiting.

"Dr. Kandelbaum, it's your turn," I said.

"Well, I'm not sure that this is the time or the place to bring this up, but I do think that it is very important for us all to think about, because it is going to affect us all, even the clinic and even the whole city, because if Wanda continues to spread HIV to everyone, then soon we'll have an epidemic of AIDS just like they have out in San Francisco, with all those people dying and everything, and it will be a public health disaster. We've got to do something for public health. I remember the measles epidemic in 1957, when we ended up quarantining all the children in the town and that stopped the epidemic. We've already tried everything else with Wanda. We taught her that 'safe sex' stuff, and gave her free condoms and the simple literature, and we did everything we know how to do, and she is still sleeping with all those men. There is no way she's telling them about her HIV status. I think that we should just quarantine her like we used to do with people with typhoid, chicken pox, and measles, so that they didn't spread the disease. I guess we could still call it "quarantine"; that's what we called it back when I was starting here, and I bet that those old rules are still on the books. It worked back then. It really cut down on those epidemics."

"Kandelbaum's right," said Weithorson. This is a public health problem and Wanda needs to be confined. Roaming around free, she's a public health menace, a regular Typhoid Mary."

"I don't think that this should have anything to do with HIV and the truckers," Jenny angrily interrupted. "If half of the truckers in this part of the state are HIV-infected," continued Jenny, "it serves them right. They pick up a girl who asks for a ride and they think that she owes them everything. If they don't know enough about safe sex, it's not because we haven't tried. There are posters in every john between here and Richardson, and condoms too. They have no right to prey on every defenseless female in the area.

"The real issue is society's treatment of those who are less fortunate. They have rights, just like everyone else, and they deserve far better than the treatment Wanda gets at the group home. The home is always asking us to prescribe sedatives and tranquilizers for the residents. All they ever seem to ask of us is for chemical restraints, drugs to do their job for them. It's much easier than teaching these poor people to be independent and to have a life of their own. The group home is paid very well to look after Wanda. I say send her back there and let them do their job properly."

"I'm worried about a legal precedent set in something called the Tarasoff case," said Goudenough, the lawyer. "It had to do with a duty to inform a potential victim. A doctor had to pay a huge settlement for not warning the victim of a patient's plan to kill her. We may have a "duty to warn." The legal precedents are tricky, but I wouldn't like to defend the case in court if some kid from a prominent family gets infected. Who is telling those truckers that playing with Wanda could kill them? I think Dr. Kandelbaum should explore public notification and the quarantine option very carefully."

Jenny was apoplectic, "With all due respect, the mentally handicapped and members of the HIV community have rights also. If anyone's concern is to avoid publicity, I think that you are doing exactly the wrong thing. I don't think you can quarantine Wanda just because she is HIV infected. You certainly can't lock her up because she is not competent to care for herself or because she's sleeping around. You've got to find some other way to control these behaviors."

Someone mumbled, "Perhaps we could ship her to Idaho."

"I'll remind you," put in the social worker, "that Medicaid regulations governing group homes require that the handicapped be kept in the 'least restrictive environment.' That means the mentally handicapped must be able to live as normal a life as possible, including the risks of everyday life. We can't pack them away so they won't hurt themselves or anyone else. The rules require that behavior may not be restricted except by the requirements of a resident's own safety, certainly not for the convenience of the caregivers or society. They go on to say something to the effect that freedom is an essential aspect of human dignity and that people with mental disabilities should be as free as anyone else in our society. We don't lock up other individuals who are HIV-positive. We urge, but don't require, that they inform their partners. What gives us the right to treat Wanda any differently?"

"Well, Doctor, I appreciate your calling this meeting," Weithorson said, "but I don't know what you expected in terms of resolving the situation. We certainly do wish, and I am sure I am speaking for all the community leaders here when I say so, that this whole thing would just go away. Please make every effort to find a nice, and most of all, secure place for Wanda. Also, work with the Department of Public Health to inform all our citizens of the dangers of AIDS. We want Wanda to have every freedom possible, within the limits of public safety, of course. Dr. Kandelbaum, you can be assured that our board and the staff of the clinic are anxious to help you in any way we can. Please feel free to call on us at any time. Thank you all for coming out at this early hour. Are there any questions? The meeting is adjourned."

* * *

Jenny grabbed two cups of coffee and joined me in my office.

"What happens now? What did that settle?" she asked.

"It looks as if we have been directed to keep out of it," I replied, "but spreading HIV infection really bothers me. In my residency, I took care of a lot of AIDS patients; it's a dreadful disease. I'm all in favor of freedom and tolerance of different life-styles and all that, so long as there is responsibility. Most of those with AIDS do act responsibly, but some don't, and it is not clear that Wanda could, even if she wanted to. What do we do then? We're back in the old conflict between the rights of the individual and those of society. I'm not sure we have ever resolved those conflicts to everyone's satisfaction.

"If we talk about the mentally handicapped, I guess we've done better. Just having group homes is huge progress compared to the old state hospitals. But are they good enough? It doesn't seem to be meeting Wanda's needs for one-on-one supervision and behavior modification. But do we have enough money to ever do all of these things? Each of these needy groups seems to be a bottomless pit. The more we provide, the more they need. How do we decide when enough is enough?

"Jenny, It's time to go back to work. Think about what you would recommend and we'll talk some more. I thought that Whiteford was going to be easy."

* * *

This case raises many ethical issues in terms of rights, duties, and virtues:

Rights

- What rights do the mentally handicapped have, even when they pose a risk to others? To what extent can Wanda be held responsible for her behavior? Is refusing to hold her responsible undercutting the human dignity that freedom is supposed to give her?
- Should the rights of HIV-positive people be limited when their actions pose a risk to others? Compare the rights of HIV-positive people with those who carry hepatitis or tuberculosis. Was quarantine of those with measles or chicken pox a justifiable curtailment of their rights? Are currently required immunizations justifiable?
- Confidentiality. Who has the right to know of Wanda's HIV status: the sheriff, the other prisoners, the other residents of the group home and their guardians, the leading citizens of Whiteford? Did the discussion of Wanda's medical situation violate the confidentiality owed to patients?

Duties

- Are community supporters of the West Whiteford Outreach Center correct to assert that the responsibilities of the clinic begin and end with the treatment of disease? If the clinic's mandate is broadened, will it lose effectiveness by trying to do too much? If the mandate is left narrow, will the clinic fail to meet many of its patients' real needs? If you believe that the clinic has social responsibilities, how extensive are they? Do they include issues of housing? poverty? family values? violence? Can health and social policy be disentangled?

- As public health authorities carry out their duty to warn the community about contagious diseases, how specific should they be in identifying the carriers of disease?

Virtues

- What constitutes a good society when it comes to the treatment of people with AIDS or mentally handicapped individuals? Will an appeal to rights advance the cause of these groups? Will an appeal to duties advance their cause?

* * *

Cases like this one do not present the same kind of alternatives as most of the other cases in this book. There is no clear course of action to be accepted or rejected. There is no key decision-maker with control of the situation. Yet cases of this kind are common in medical practice. They occupy the border between care for individual patients and the responsibility of physicians for community health and public policy.

What is your response to the issues raised in this case? If you were in this physician's place, what would you do about Wanda?

chapter
7

* * * * *

The Maxistop Study

"Well the worst that can happen is they pee in their pants. People don't literally die of embarrassment," smirked the chief resident sliding into her chair, late as usual, for the meeting of the Institutional Review Board of St. Catherine Hospital.

"That's not a great way to start this meeting off," responded Dr. John Boston.

"If you'll pardon the expression, the whole thing smells bad to me. Why are we messing with this anyway?" put in Dr. Barbara Rowe, physician and activist.

The always patient Dr. Boston, director of the family practice outreach clinic and chairman of the IRB, heaved one of his customary sighs and continued: "University Hospital upstate has offered us an opportunity to participate in a research study of Maxistop. They hope this new drug will be an improved treatment for urinary incontinence, a major embarrassment for a lot of older women. One of their professors has a big contract from Sonarch Pharmaceuticals. They need us to recruit patients for their study.

"Federal regulations require that our IRB committee review the design of the study and especially the informed-consent materials. Although the people at University have already gone over it, we have to do the same thing. That's why we have this 50-page study document to review. If we don't approve the research, it doesn't happen here."

The Research Plan

"So what if it doesn't happen here? What's in it for us?" put in the chief resident.

"Actually, a number of small but good things come with this project. The elderly women we enrol get an extra-thorough workup at the beginning of the study and a follow-up check six months later—all paid for. We might pick up something serious on one or two of them. The subjects get the experimental drug free, $100 to show up for the second visit, and a year's supply of the drug if it works for them.

"The clinic gets $500 for every patient we enrol; that's to cover our expenses. If we recruit 50 patients, we could get a new x-ray machine that would really help us out. It will also get the residents into some research. I know it's not rocket science, but even this kind of research will be stimulating for them. It shows we're not just stuck out here in the boonies pushing pills. Also, for icing on the cake, the residents get 2,500 frequent flier miles for every patient they sign up."

"Let me see if I'm clear about the study design," said Professor Lombardo, a biochemist at the local branch of the state university. "This is a placebo-controlled, double-blinded clinical trial. The double blind part makes sense. Urinary incontinence may well have a psychological component, so the patient should not know whether she is getting the medicine or only an inert pill. Also, the people dealing with the patient should not know either because they could, unconsciously of course, give signals to the patient.

"But why is this a placebo trial? Isn't there anything on the market for this condition?"

"There are several drugs out there," responded Dr. Boston, "but none of them work terribly well. Sonarch hopes this drug will be an improvement, but it may not be a great leap forward. If we compare this drug with an available drug, it may not show a statistically significant difference. It's much easier to show that a drug is 'safe and effective' against a placebo. Besides, everyone calls a placebo trial the 'gold standard' of research; the Food and Drug Administration (FDA) typically wants this kind of study."

"I'm beginning to have a problem here," put in Dr. Rowe. "Why are we asking these women to take a chance on getting a sugar pill when there is something available that we know can help them? A placebo trial make sense when we have nothing else to offer, but not when there are other drugs available. Are we taking advantage of them because of their gender and age?

"I don't see that this drug offers any benefit to our patients. Why are we looking to participate in the study? I believe that it is all about greed. Sonarch wants to market a drug that can compete with the three other incontinence medications out there. They have been quite profitable for the drug companies because incontinence is an issue for elderly women. These women are usually on Medicare and it pays for the drugs. Each drug has been shown to be somewhat better—statistically—than placebo, so it passes the FDA's effectiveness test. None of them are very effective, but at least none of them are very harmful. So they are marketed, at quite high prices, and Medicare pays for everything except the deductible. But the company, in its eagerness and greed to get into the trough, is not the only hungry one in this story.

"What is the hospital's interest? The hospital never had an interest in research until Sonarch waved a bunch of money under its nose. It smells the potential for geriatric patients with other medical problems. It sees income from these patients in the clinic, and the possibility of a new x-ray machine. Perhaps even further research contracts if it is a good recruiter of patients. The residents are paid in frequent flyer miles and you think they will learn how to do research for other drug companies. What they'll actually learn is how to accept invitations to fancy dinner meetings where they'll learn how to recruit patients. There will be trips to exotic places to learn about the drug and to spread the word of its substantial wonders compared to placebos.

"I don't think there is a shred of scientific value in this study. Everyone in this room knows the outcome of the study right now. The drug is probably safe. It will be just like all of the other marginally effective drugs. And we will document this at the expense of these poor old ladies, half of whom will get a sugar pill instead of the currently available medications.

"This is merely another 'me-too' drug. Sonarch is probably marketing a minor variation on something already out there. This study is more about marketing than serious medical research. I'd be ashamed to vote in favor of participating in the study."

"That's not quite accurate, Barbara," responded Dr. Boston. "The principal investigator is an old friend. She tells me the experimental drug is not chemically similar to the other drugs for incontinence. Instead, it's a chemical relative of compounds that have been around a long time for the treatment of seasonal allergies. University has done the Phase I and Phase II studies, the toxicity and safety trials. We can be sure we're not going to kill anyone with this stuff. She assures me we have no need to worry about the side effects.

"Also, there are a lot of other hospitals that would like to get in on this research. If we don't approve it, they will. If we start acting holier-than-thou, University and the drug companies will just take their research contracts elsewhere. I had to plead to get this study. If we turn it down, nobody but us will suffer."

* * *

As medicine has firmly established its scientific base, the controlled clinical trial has become the standard for medical research. It provides physicians with solidly established scientific knowledge on which to base their decisions. Good design of clinical trials is a very complex scientific matter, and even well-designed trials can raise significant ethical problems.

Unfortunately, the history of human experimentation in medicine is replete with ethical problems. From the gross violations of human beings that marked the Nazi medical experiments to the radiation and syphillis studies in the United States, research subjects have been physically abused, deceived, and subjected to unknown risks, all without their knowledge much less their consent. These ethical violations have scarred biomedical research.

In an effort to prevent further violations, the U.S. Food and Drug Administration requires that clinical trials and other research with human subjects be approved by institutional review boards, the local committees at each institution participating in the trial. Other federal agencies, such as the National Institutes of Health and the National Institutes of Mental Health, as well as leading medical journals, have similar requirements.

The study discussed in this case presents some of the ethical problems typically faced by IRBs:

Placebo Design.   Is a placebo design ethically acceptable when there is an approved therapy available? Many trials compare a new therapy against an established one, but the FDA "gold standard" is the placebo-controlled trial. Since good results appear more clearly against a placebo background, such trials actually make it easier to introduce new medicines. Is a placebo design acceptable in this case because the implications of drug failure are not severe? Wetting one's pants, after all, is only an embarrassment and an inconvenience. Would the study be acceptable if Maxistop were an anti-cancer drug or a contraceptive? Would you participate in a placebo-controlled trial of a contraceptive?

How effective would the available drugs have to be before you would object to a placebo-controlled trial? If the best available drug were 90 percent effective in dealing with the condition, would you object to a placebo trial? What if it were 10 percent effective? If your answer is somewhere in the middle, where and how do you draw that line? On the other hand, if the FDA wants a placebo trial, is that good enough for you?

Me-Too Studies.   Some drug company research is devoted to "me-too" drugs, minor variants of effective drugs designed to give companies a share the lucrative market for widely used medications. Would you object to this study solely on the ground that it is a me-too study? Would the study be invalid if it gave no new scientific information but gave the drug company access to a new market, did not harm participants, and provided some other benefits to those who conducted and those who participated in the study? People participate in marketing research all the time, sometimes for a lot less reward than these patients will receive. If patients give their informed consent and even get some rewards for their participation, does it make a difference that the research is more directed at marketing and sales than at science?

Incentives for Patients and Researchers.   Some critics view such incentives as bribery, or at least as compromising the freedom of patients to refuse to participate in clinical trials. Will the incentives offered to the patients in this study distort their ability to make a free and informed decision about participating in the trial? Should these incentives be eliminated? Or are the study subjects undercompensated in light of the incentives for those conducting the study and the potential profits for Sonarch?

The physicians who would be recruiting the study's subjects are the primary care physicians for these patients. Are they single-mindedly devoted to their patients' care, or would they become double agents, working also for the drug company? Should all these patients be getting an "extra-thorough" physical exam as part of their routine care? Why do they need to participate in a study in order to get one? Does the promise of frequent flier miles distort physicians' judgment about what is good for their patients? Does the prospect of improved x-ray equipment distort the judgment of the clinic's director about what is good for the patients and the residents?

Does the friendship between the clinic's director and the principal investigator compromise the IRB's independence?

Informed Consent

Would the adequate informed consent of the study participants eliminate the above objections to the proposed study? Consider that the findings of the Nuremberg trials established informed consent as the critical factor in the conduct of ethically acceptable human experiments (see Chapter 19). Is free and informed consent a sufficient test of the moral acceptability of a human research study?

"Our prime responsibility is review of the informed consent document," continued Dr. Boston. "That's the heart of our responsibility. We respect our patients' autonomy so long as they know what we are about and freely consent to participate in the experiment. They should be free to participate, and equally free to turn us down. That's how I understand the standard that the Nuremberg Commission established. Just as placebo trials are the FDA's gold standard, free and informed consent is the ethical gold standard.

"Let's review the proposed consent form; it's in the back of your booklet."

Informed Consent to Participate in a Clinical Trial of Iridium Sulfate (*Maxistop*) for Urinary Incontinence

Before you agree to participate voluntarily as one of 3,000 patients in this study of the treatment of urinary incontinence, it is important that you read and understand the following explanation of the proposed procedures. The purpose of this study is to compare the frequency and severity of incontinent events between two treatment groups. One treatment group will receive *Maxistop* to be taken twice daily, the other group will receive placebo (inactive substance). *Maxistop* is in a class of drugs widely used to treat rhinitis. It acts as a beta channel agonist, blockading neuronal pathways to the genitourinary anatomy. You will be randomized in this study, which means that neither you nor your physician will know whether you are in the control or the *Maxistop* group. The study will take about six months. You may withdraw from it at any time without jeopardizing your relationship with your physician or St. Catherine Hospital. We only ask that you state in writing your reasons for so doing. If you agree to participate in this study, you will receive two thorough physical examinations, fifty dollars at the second examination, and a one year supply of *Maxistop* at the conclusion of the study (if it is successful). You will not be charged for the examinations or for the medications used in the study. Neither St. Catherine Hospital nor your physician, however, are responsible for any adverse events that may be connected with this study. We offer no assurance that we will cover the treatment of untoward events. If you have any questions now or in the course of the study, you may contact Sonarch Pharmaceutical's help line at (800) 555-1212.

"It's all pretty standard stuff," continued Dr. Boston. "They all sound alike after a while. Let's go down our check sheet to make sure everything's covered."

IRB Checksheet—Review of Informed Consent

Is the form readable by the patients likely to be enrolled in the study? Does the consent form explain:

That it is a research study?

The purpose of the study?

The length of subject's participation?

Description of procedures?

Identification of experimental procedures?

Description of risks to subject?

Description of benefits of the research to subject or others?

Alternative treatments?

Confidentiality of records and the fact that the FDA may inspect records?

Availability of treatment if injuries occur and where information may be obtained?

Contacts for questions concerning research patient's rights?

Voluntary participation—refusal to participate results in no loss of benefits to patient?

Discontinuation at any time without loss of benefits?

Conditions under which researchers may drop patient from the study?

Costs to the subject?

Notification of significant findings that may affect subject's willingness to continue?

"Any problems here?" continued Dr. Boston. "What do you say?"

* * *

Take your place as a member of this IRB and think of how you might respond to Dr. Rowe's charges. Is she being holier-than-thou? Is she guilty of moral absolutism when the situation calls for a pragmatic attitude? Begin by looking at the nature of the research.

Does the research seem to offer sufficient benefits in relation to whatever the risks it poses to the research subjects? If you believe there is no great scientific value to this research, is it morally acceptable as marketing research? Should marketing research be held to a different ethical standard than clinical research?

Are the incentives for participants and researchers appropriate? Will subjects be coerced into the trial by unduly large rewards to the researchers? How large should the rewards be? Could they be larger than those mentioned in this study and still be acceptable?

Follow the check sheet step-by-step. Does the proposed informed consent form meet its requirements? Are all these requirements reasonable? If the list of requirements is reasonable but the consent form is not adequate, what would the researchers need to add or to change in the form?

On completing this review, would you approve the Maxistop study? How would you respond to Dr. Rowe's objections?

Would you recommend that your mother participate in this study?

CHILDHOOD AND ADOLESCENCE

chapter

8

* * * * *

Joey, Jessica, Roger, Tom, and Marti

AUTHORS' NOTE: *Although we present this case with pediatric patients, the main issue it raises—the allocation of scarce medical resources or rationing—has no special connection with this population.*

It is a beautiful Memorial Day weekend, which means trouble for you. As a fellow in intensive care medicine at University Hospital, you know it is going to be tough. There will be automobile accidents, boating accidents, plus all the usual problems. Since University provides the highest level of pediatric intensive care in the entire state, you know you will be busy.

Indeed, as you sign in with the ICU ward clerk at 8 A.M. on Saturday, you see from the patient board that every bed is occupied. This means that even at the beginning of the weekend you are on "flyby." The helicopters that bring injured children to major medical centers now have an order to bypass University for the less well equipped regional centers. The regional centers are not bad; they can handle 90 percent of the cases. However, there is that 10 percent that only the staff and facilities at University can handle really well.

You are especially concerned about the victims of near-drownings. University has a special project in this area, and you and the residents and nurses with whom you work have developed into a team for handling these cases. The team has had excellent results. Children who would have died elsewhere walk out of University with minimal damage. The outcome from many other centers may even be worse—an irreversible coma preceding a lingering death. Although not many people will be swimming today, there will be a lot of boating on the lake. The water is still cold, and that is good for preserving brain function. If some children were to get in trouble, you would have an excellent chance of helping them.

You join the rest of the team in the conference room and begin a review of the patients. Most of the review is just the daily update on each patient's condition. But you and the rest of the staff are anxious to see if one or two patients could be moved out to make room for any disaster that might happen. Here are the patients that at least one member of the staff thinks are good candidates for leaving the ICU.

Joey

Joey is the 7-year-old kid wearing the Milwaukee Brewers cap and "sleeping" peacefully in the far corner of room B. Joey has been that way for six months now, and he will never wake up. His brain was severely damaged when his mother's boyfriend, in a drunken stupor, knocked him around the room. The resulting skull fracture and concussion built up such pressure in his head that most of the blood flow through his brain was cut off. His entire cortex, the seat of all the higher functions of the brain, was destroyed by the lack of oxygen. Only a few of his brainstem functions remain. He withdraws from deep pain; if his upper arm muscles are pinched hard, he tries to pull away. His pupils narrow when a light is shined in his eyes. If a cotton swab is brushed across the back of his throat, he gags. He exerts some effort to breathe, but he is now on a respirator because he does not exert enough respiratory effort to sustain himself. If he were disconnected from the respirator, he would gasp for air and shortly die.

This will be Joey's fate. His mother was unwilling to accept it for a long time, especially because the charge against her boyfriend will be changed from assault to murder. Slowly and grudgingly she has come to see that Joey's condition is incurable and that the respirator is merely keeping him breathing. The Child Abuse Agency of the Department of Social Services finally accepted it as well, reluctantly agreeing to get a court order to allow University to discontinue useless therapy; as Joey's guardians, no decision could be made without them, and they took a long time making up their minds. Because Joey's injury is the basis for a criminal prosecution, the district attorney also had to approve withdrawing the respirator. She took only a week to decide that withdrawing the respirator would not damage her case for a murder conviction.

It had taken three months to stabilize Joey's condition and to be sure that he had suffered irreversible brain damage. It took the second three months to put the pieces of a decision together. Just this past Wednesday, everyone involved had been in court reviewing the entire case before Judge McBrien. He heard everyone out, asked a number of questions of the physicians about how sure they were that Joey would not recover (they were very sure), and announced that he would hand down his decision in a week. The hospital's attorneys assured the ICU team that there would be no problem; Judge McBrien would let them withdraw the respirator. They cautioned, however, that the judge did not like being rushed and that he liked his weekends off. There was nothing to do, the attorneys advised, but wait one more week.

Joey's fate, then, was decided, but you are powerless to do anything about it. If you turn the respirator off before the judge hands down his order, you and the hospital could be guilty of contempt of court. Worse, you would never again get a sympathetic hearing from Judge McBrien or other judges if you needed a decision in a similar case.

The only other possibility is to move Joey to another ward in the hospital. But there are problems here as well. Hospital policy is very clear on the point: no pediatric respirator patients outside the ICU. The policy is based on some bad past experiences. Furthermore, since the staff on other wards has lost touch with the care of respirator patients, there is the risk that Joey might die outside the ICU. That might not sit well with the judge, and who knows what effect it would have on the prosecution of Joey's assailant.

As you run through these considerations with the team, there is a growing sense of frustration and anger. Who are we treating, they ask, Joey or the lawyers? We did absolutely everything we could for Joey, and it did not work. For the last three months, all we have been doing is warehousing him while everyone goes to meetings. Now we may find ourselves in the position of keeping Joey in the ICU while turning away some child we could really help. This is an abuse of everything the ICU stands for; it is immoral unless we can free up Joey's bed or some other bed in the ICU. You agree, but what can you do? You go on to the next case.

Jessica

Jessica, like Joey, will soon be out of the ICU, but her story will have a happy ending. She is a 12-year-old with Guillain-Barre syndrome, an inflammation of the nervous system that sometimes follows a viral infection. The disease causes a progressive paralysis, starting in the hands and feet and proceeding to the trunk. It is usually self-limiting and self-reversing. In 90 percent of the cases, the disease is not recurrent and there are no long-term effects. When the disease affects the trunk, however, the muscles of the chest become paralyzed and the patient cannot breathe on her own. These patients are placed on respirators until their nerve functions return and their muscles regain normal strength.

Jessica has been in the ICU for about two weeks, and she is doing very well. The paralysis seems to be improving, and she is starting to recover. Her respiratory muscles have not regained full strength, so she still needs some support from a respirator. It will be about two weeks before she can be taken off it entirely.

As in Joey's case, hospital policy requires that Jessica stay in the ICU.

Unlike Joey's, the quality of medical care will have a bearing on the outcome of her case. If someone on another ward makes a mistake in handling Jessica, even though it would be difficult to make such a mistake because her care is relatively simple at this point, Jessica could suffer brain damage. The nurse who has been working most closely with Jessica is adamant.

"There is no way Jessica is going anywhere else. I know she doesn't need a great deal of care at this moment, but no one else in this hospital is truly competent to provide that care. It would simply be immoral to transfer Jessica to another ward. We can't take that chance on a child who is doing so well.

"Furthermore, if you want to talk hospital policy and legal problems, what kind of shape would we be in if something happened to Jessica? Her father is a lawyer, and he was very upset when their local pediatrician didn't make the diagnosis right away. If we try anything less than standard medical care, all hell will break loose."

The resident in charge of the near-drowning resuscitation group now spoke up.

"It just isn't true that Jessica's care off this ward would be substandard. The hospital's policy on respirator patients is very artificial, especially in a case like this when Jessica doesn't require that much. We even send kids home on respirators. It is crazy that we can't send them to another unit in this hospital. We would have to hunt up a nurse with some respirator experience, or even send one of you down to check on things, but Jessica will do just fine. In the meantime, we would be able to help someone for whom the ICU is a life-or-death matter. Right now Jessica requires chronic care. She is not really an intensive care patient. We don't have to move her before we have another patient, of course, but I think she is the logical one to go if the need arises."

In Joey's case, the team had been pretty much of one mind. The ICU was not doing anything for Joey, but the legal risks of moving him out were very high. In Jessica's case, there was a division of opinion among the staff, so you thought it best to move on.

Roger

Roger is dead. He committed suicide on Thursday night by putting his father's revolver in his mouth and firing. From the time he was brought to the emergency room, it was clear there was no hope. It was also clear that he was an ideal organ donor. Fifteen-year-old Roger was placed on a respirator immediately and treated to insure the survival of his heart, kidneys, liver, and other transplantable organs. The neurology resident examined him on Friday and agreed that all clinical signs said that Roger was dead. He had no gag reflex, made no effort to breath when temporarily disconnected from the respirator, and made no response to pain. A test of brain waves (electroencephalogram

[EEG]) showed a tiny amount of activity. A second test ordered for today will undoubtedly show no activity. The neurologists will declare Roger dead whenever you want.

Yesterday was very hard. Roger's parents are completely devastated. The nurses and a psychiatrist spent all day yesterday with them. Although Roger had previously shown signs of what is now recognized as depression, he had no prior history of mental illness and had never threatened suicide. His parents slowly and painfully came to accept Roger's death and even raised the possibility of his being an organ donor. It was a way that some part of him would remain alive; even in death he would make some contribution. They signed the papers last evening.

Meanwhile, the hospital's own transplant group was alerted. After doing blood and tissue typing on Roger, they identified him as a heart donor for one of their patients. The liver transplant team in a nearby state was notified, and they had a suitable recipient. They were gearing up, and a group would fly in late today to pick up Roger's liver. The kidney transplant group was also preparing two recipients.

The plan was to take Roger to an operating room in the early evening. He would be declared dead, the respirator would be removed, and the organs would be taken for transplant. Until then, Roger would stay on the respirator and on his blood pressure medications to keep his organs in shape. Nothing could be done before early evening because it would take at least that long for the transplant teams to get ready.

"I think Roger is the one who should go," says the head nurse. "He's dead. He is no longer a patient. No matter what shape the others are in, they are our patients and we are committed to doing what is best for them, even if, in Joey's case, it means doing little or nothing. These transplant patients are not ours. It will be a shame if they do not get Roger's organs, but that's not our problem. We have to keep our eyes on what we're doing here, not looking out for everyone else's problems."

"That's a good point," volunteered the resident who was directing the near-drowning project; another resident reminded the group that the people coming in on helicopters aren't their patients either.

"Not exactly right," the nurse replied. "We have a special state grant to operate the near-drowning resuscitation program. We've trained the helicopter crews. Once drowning victims are picked up, they are our patients. As part of the state program, we have a responsibility for them."

You raise the point that the team may have a responsibility to Roger, even though he is dead. Yesterday you made a commitment to accept his organs for donation. That means a lot to his parents and might even mean something to him had he been aware of it. Besides, you add, perhaps the crunch will not come until tomorrow after all the organ donations have taken place.

"Could we at least transfer him to pediatrics temporarily?" asks one of the residents.

"Not if you're serious about maintaining his organs in decent shape for the next 6 to 8 hours," responds the head nurse. "With all Roger's drugs and machines—no way those nurses could handle that. Managing organs for transplant is as tricky as any work we do on this unit. We're already short-staffed on the holiday. He needs constant monitoring to keep his blood pressure up. It will take the full-time attention of one of our best nurses."

"Is there any way we could go over census and squeeze an extra bed in here?" you ask.

"The space, the bed, and the equipment are not the problem," the head nurse explains. "The hospital is always ready to spend money on hardware. Until the last few years, we had people on call, and we could count on finding experienced staff for an emergency. But in the last couple of years those guys with the pointy pencils and heads to match have been running the hospital; 'lean and mean' they like to say. They've cut nursing to the bone. Lots of the experienced nurses have quit, leaving with a real sour taste for the place. We just don't have any reserve of the kind of help we need.

"Of course I can call one of the temp agencies, but their people aren't ready for the kind of high-tech nursing problems we're facing this weekend. On top of that, Nancy called in sick. We'll be lucky to get by as it is," says the head nurse.

Your mental list of candidates for non-ICU treatment is exhausted, and you are about to get a cup of coffee and think the thing through when Karen, the pediatric resident, interrupts.

"I think you are skipping over two of the most obvious players," she says. "There are two kids here with chronic conditions that, in my view, are better nominees than any of the three we've been talking about.

"I took an ethics course in college," she continues, "and we talked about cases like this in terms of the allocation of scarce medical resources. It was a question of social ethics and public policy. Our discussion is looking at individual cases too narrowly, taking them out of their social context. The three cases we've talked about so far will be over in a day, or maybe a week. But there are two kids in this unit who have long-term, massive, and very expensive problems. I think we should consider moving them out of the unit because I don't think it's right for society to treat them. For what it's costing to treat these two kids, we could do near-drowning cases for a decade. I'm thinking of Tom and Marti."

Tom

Tom was born about 18 months ago with prune-belly syndrome. Just before the midpoint of his mother's pregnancy, his urethra became blocked and the urine backed up into his bladder and then into the kidneys. This condition was detected in an ultrasound exam at about the 26th week of pregnancy, and his mother was referred to the obstetrical group at University. Tom's mother was in her middle 30s, a professional woman who had long postponed having a child. Amniocentesis showed Tom to be genetically normal, and she was anxious for any help to continue the pregnancy. In turn, the obstetrical group was anxious to get started on new techniques of in-utero surgery. They persuaded Tom's mother to let them try.

In the 28th week of the pregnancy, the obstetrical surgeons inserted a catheter through his mother's abdomen into Tom's distended bladder. This shunt drained urine from the bladder into the amniotic fluid, decompressing the kidneys and restoring the normal amniotic fluid volume.

It was one of those "the operation was a success but the patient died" stories, only this patient did not die. Tom was born in the 34th week of his mother's pregnancy. The pressure on his kidneys was relieved only temporarily. As the volume of amniotic fluid again declined because the shunt stopped working, Tom's mother started premature labor. The obstetricians decided that an early delivery would give Tom the best chance, so they did a Caesarean section.

Tom was born with a grossly distended, wrinkly abdomen—hence the name "prune-belly" syndrome. In addition, as is common in this condition, his lungs were underdeveloped. Tom was placed on a respirator at birth and, despite several attempts, his underdeveloped lungs have frustrated every effort to wean him from the machine.

Over the past 18 months, everything was tried, and nothing worked very well. The damage that Tom's lungs suffered in utero could not be significantly reversed, nor could the kidney damage be reversed, so Tom needs regular dialysis. Moreover, Tom has not done well intellectually or socially. His development has been substantially slow, although there is no clear reason for this. Tom's mother has stuck with him, but it is now clear that he is not developing normally.

"Listen," Karen argued, "we all know now that the obstetricians made a mistake. They never should have tried their fancy new operation; they were just hopping on the bandwagon. Even in the literature then available, there was good reason to think it wouldn't work. But once we got started, no one has been able to say 'stop.' Tom is stable, of course, but none of us is facing the fact that he will never come off the respirator and that he will never lead what remotely could be called a normal life. His development is very poor, and it isn't going to get any better. I think we should take him off the respirator and let him die."

There was a commotion around the room, and someone said, "We can't do that!"

When the hubbub died down, Karen continued, "That's the whole trouble with these chronic care kids. There is rarely so severe a crisis that we're forced to face up to their troubles. We have been mumbling things to Tom's mother, but we've never sat down to confront her with the facts and, worst of all, we've never confronted ourselves with the facts. There never is a good time to make these decisions. We've already made the decision, but we're just not facing it. We talk about weaning him off the respirator, and we know that's faking it. He'll never make it. Somehow or other, we're going to cut back and he's going to die. Let's cut our losses and act now. We have to admit that our very expensive therapy hasn't worked, and we can no longer afford to keep Tom going, especially because he is going nowhere."

Karen has a good case, and you know it. But you just do not see how the issue can be so finally resolved this weekend. You ask Karen to mention the other case she has in mind. "The other patient we should discontinue treatment on is Marti."

Marti

From a medical point of view, Marti's case is simple and tragic. A 14-year-old, she was riding in her mother's car when it stopped at a light and was rear-ended at high speed by a drunk driver. Marti's spinal cord was severed at the C2 level, the very top of the neck. Essentially, in terms of control, Marti's head was severed from the rest of her body. She is a quadraplegic—completely paralyzed from the neck down and, therefore, breathes only because she is on a respirator. She is unable to move her legs, arms, or head. She talks, of course, and her intellectual ability is unaffected.

Marti has been in intensive care for about three months. The initial purpose of her stay was to stabilize her condition and to be sure that the spinal cord damage was complete and irreversible. Now she remains in the ICU awaiting transfer to a rehabilitation hospital.

The driver of the car that hit her had no insurance and no assets to help pay for Marti's care. Marti's father is between jobs; her mother spends all her time caring for her. They have minimal insurance. Marti's care is now being handled by the state fund for crippled children.

"This is going to sound awful," Karen said, "but I think it is unfair to keep Marti alive at overwhelming expense when that same money could be used to help so many people. The level of medical care she will require is more than society should invest in any one person. In most places in the world, she would have died soon after the accident. We've assessed her condition, and we know just how handicapped she is going to be. This sounds very hard, but we should sedate her and pull the plug."

"Today?" you ask.

"We could send her down to pediatrics," says one of the residents.

"Unlike Jessica," you reply, "she is totally dependent on the respirator. There's a terrible risk sending her down to the ward; she couldn't survive even the slightest glitch."

Karen's previous proposal had caused a commotion; this one caused a near riot. People were shouting and pounding the table. It just showed how attached they'd become to this totally dependent girl. "What kind of morality is that, Karen?" asks one of the other residents. "You'd turn off the respirator on someone with normal intelligence just because she's physically handicapped?"

"I suppose there's the alternative of moving Tom or Marti down to the ward," you add, "but that still poses the respirator problems. Next week we should discuss long-term plans for them. Now is the time to get back to work and to hope that the roof doesn't fall in." You head for the door still hoping that you won't have to make any decisions.

Later That Morning

Several hours later the call comes. You are talking with Marti, who is very depressed. She doesn't want to see the psychiatrist any more, and she thinks it would have been better if she had died in the accident. The soccer season is just ending, and her team lost in the finals. "I'll never be able to do anything," she wheezes around the tracheotomy tube in her throat.

Sally, the triage nurse, pages you to the red phone. As you come down the hall, she calls out that it is Mike from the state police rescue unit. He is on a dock in Lake City with two kids who have just been rescued. The red phone connects you directly with him in the helicopter.

"Hey, Doc, you have to make room for these kids. They're great candidates for you. Their boat tipped over and they were only under water for about ten minutes. They are brothers, 7 and 9 years old. Some guys in another boat saw them go in, fished them out, and did some CPR. Both are breathing but cold and unconscious. I radioed Lakeside Community Hospital right away because I knew you were on flyby. Lakeside pleaded with me to have you take them. They have plenty of room but nobody competent with near-drowning. I wanted to take a look at the kids and size up the situation, the way you trained us, before calling in. This is a great setup for your new treatments, but sending them to Lakeside is signing their death warrants, or worse. You just have to take these kids, Doc."

* * *

You've been over all of the other alternatives and there just aren't any. The only way you could take one or both of the boys is by displacing one or two of your ICU patients.

If you decide to take one or both of the boys, you have about two hours to decide who to displace and to make appropriate arrangements. You can evaluate and stabilize the drowning victims in the emergency room, but within two hours there will have to be room in your ICU.

Think carefully about your tentative decision and the justification for your choice. If you decide to displace one or more of the children from the ICU, also think about why you didn't select the others.

* * *

Reconsidering and Justifying Your Decision

The best and safest thing for each of the ICU patients is to remain in the ICU. Unfortunately, that is also the best place for the boys on the dock. For each child there is an increased risk if they are removed from the ICU or not brought there. How did you balance the risks and benefits in making your decision?

Ethical theory provides guidelines for making these decisions. Different theories use different bases. Here are a few.

Quality of Individual Life

Which patients gain the most from being in the ICU? Who will lose the most by being moved out? Who will lose the least? Does Roger have anything to lose? What about Joey and Tom? How about Jessica and Marti? Rank the five patients in order of who has the most to lose. Is that a moral basis for deciding who should stay? Where did you rank the boys on the dock? How much do we know about what they have to lose?

Social Utility

Should you look beyond what an individual has to gain or lose and include family, other individuals, and society in your calculations? This is called social benefit analysis, a type of utilitarian theory.

Social benefit analysis tries to add up the total happiness of the individual and the happiness of all those with whom he is associated and affects. For example, an anencephalic, an infant with no brain, has no capability for experiencing happiness or satisfaction. If he brings no joy to those around him, he has no social utility. If his family derives some pleasure from him, then he has some utility.

Using this type of calculation, rank the children in the ICU.

How did you rank Roger? Does the fact that he is dead imply that he has no individual utility? What about his social utility to the organ recipients? Does this raise his utility above that of Joey? Tom? Jessica? How would you rank Jessica's utility, when she will be a perfectly normal child, against what Roger can accomplish for several others? How about Marti? What is her "utility" score? How many points do you give her for happiness? Is her depression a transient state?

Now give a score to the boys on the dock. Where do they fit into your rank order? Do you know enough about them? You don't even know enough to guess at their prognosis. Will they end up like Joey? Or like Jessica? Write down your rankings of the seven individuals.

Rights and Obligations

Under rights and obligations theory, there are certain inalienable rights with which an individual is born. Among these are the right to respect as a person, from which may flow the right to life or at least the right not to be killed; the right to liberty, often used in the political sense, but also including the right to control of one's own person and one's medical care. While many philosophers articulate rights in different fashions and while even the preceding three rights overlap and flow from one another, they are basic rights of personhood.

We are born with some rights, and others are acquired by the commitments and contracts made by other individuals in society. The right to vote, for example, is given by the state and may be withdrawn, as with felons, or extended, as it was to 18-year-olds. The right to medical care is a source of debate, but in our society it often flows from a contract or commitment between patient and physician.

Are rights absolute and equal? Or do they have varying degrees of magnitude? Can you rank the patients in order of their rights? Does Roger have any rights? Do the transplant recipients have any rights? Does Joey have any rights? Are Joey's rights just legal and not moral? Are moral rights stronger or weaker than legal rights?

Do the boys on the dock have a right to your care? Is that right greater than that of any of the ICU patients? If so, what will you do about it?

Now list these same patients in terms of the strength of your obligation to each. Do you have an obligation to the boys on the dock? Do you have an obligation to Roger, even though he is dead? Do you have an obligation to Roger's parents, to the transplant teams, and to the potential transplant recipients? Are your obligations to the transplant teams affected by the commitment that your hospital has made to the transplant program? After you have ranked the patients in terms of the strength of your obligations, compare that list with the other lists you have prepared. How are they related to each other? Which list should be used to make a moral decision?

Now make your decision. How will you handle this crisis? Although you have time to carry out your decision, you have little time to actually decide.

Not only is what you do important, but why you do it counts as well. How have you justified your decision? Later events may require that you look back at this first decision, and it will be important to remember why you decided as you did.

1. If you decided to turn down one or both boys, go to the section entitled "You Turn Down the Drowning Victims."
2. If you have decided to displace Joey, you had better discuss this with Judge McBrien first. Read "Joey" immediately following.
3. If you plan to displace Jessica, at least call her father and tell him why you changed your mind about keeping her in the ICU. Then go to the section entitled "Jessica."
4. If you plan to displace Roger, call his parents. They were waiting to hear from you about the transplants. Go to "Roger."
5. If you plan to displace Marti, Tom, or both go to "Marti or Tom."
6. If you decide to accept both boys, decide whom to displace and follow the decision to its end; then return to this page and decide on the second displacement.

Joey

After a lengthy effort you finally locate Judge McBrien at his cottage on the lake. The state police found the boat on which he was fishing. The judge does not take kindly to having his weekend disturbed.

You outline the problem to the judge and carefully explain why it is important to turn off Joey's respirator now. Other lives are at stake.

With seeming patience, the judge explains that he has been thinking deeply about the case and that he thinks best when he is on the lake and undisturbed. "This is not an easy case," he says. "You realize, of course, that Joey is not brain dead. By legal standards, if you turn off the respirator you will be killing him. I am agonizing over this case because I don't like my cases appealed and my decisions overturned. I'll let you know my final decision on Wednesday. Please don't disturb me again."

* * *

If, in the face of your discussion with Judge McBrien, you decide that you better not do anything about Joey, turn back to the list of options and choose again.

If you decide that, even though you can't turn off the respirator, you can transfer Joey to pediatrics and take a chance, then continue.

* * *

You transfer Joey to pediatrics and discuss the case with the residents and nurses there. You emphasize the need for careful monitoring and tell them to call you with any questions or problems. At 1 A.M. Sunday, Joey's respirator became disconnected. The alarm on the machine did not function. At 2 A.M., when the nurse came in to check his vital signs, Joey was dead.

At noon on Sunday, you are called to the offices of the hospital's general counsel. They are not happy about spending Sunday at work and are getting ready to go to court tomorrow to break the news to Judge McBrien. They are preparing a memorandum to the judge explaining why the issues placed before him are now moot.

They ask you to prepare a brief explanation of what happened to Joey and why he was chosen to be removed from the ICU. Incorporate the considerations you made regarding patients' rights and your obligations to your patients as well as any considerations of risk, benefits, and consequences. Also acknowledge any obligations you have to the courts, the legal systems, and Judge McBrien. After you've finished your explanation, go to "Conclusion," at the end of this chapter.

Jessica

You locate Jessica's father in Chicago, where he is working with a client. He comes to the phone breathlessly.

"Is there something wrong? When I left last night Jessica really seemed so much better and happier, we were really beginning to be hopeful. What happened?"

You reassure him that nothing has happened, that you are calling because she is doing so well. You explain about the near-drownings and the need for room in the ICU. Jessica is clearly making a good recovery. "I am planning to move her and her respirator down to pediatrics. She should do just fine. We'll put her right across from the nurses' station so they can watch her just in case anything happens."

"What do you mean, in case? What could happen? You told me she needs to be in the ICU another two weeks because it was the safest place for someone on a respirator."

After much discussion and as much reassurance as you can muster, Jessica's father acquiesces with one condition. "Dr. Dunn is an old friend of mine from high school days. He is chief of pediatrics. I know he would look out for her best interests. If he says it's okay, I guess it will be. I'll be in to see her when I get back tomorrow."

You put down the phone and call Dr. Dunn, whose wife tells you that he has just left for an international congress in Germany. "Can I help? Dr. Dunn has left that nice young man, Brian, in charge. Why don't you try him?"

Your friend Brian is chief resident in pediatrics. You call him; his response is just what you would expect. "I feel for you, buddy. Two near-drowning victims and such a beautiful weekend; you'll never get out for tennis. Sure we'll take her. I'll square it with our head nurse. She doesn't mind bending the rules a bit. Sounds like Jessica shouldn't be a problem. It's a good thing Dunn's out of town—he's pretty rigid about those things. I'll be on the courts if you can get away."

* * *

If you decide to take Brian's offer, continue reading this section. But if you are concerned about not getting Dr. Dunn's permission, as Jessica's father had insisted, go back to the list of options and choose again.

* * *

Jessica came out of it fine; you are confident that she suffered no permanent damage. But Dr. French, the chief of Critical Care Medicine, is standing there with a blank incident report form. You had Jessica moved to pediatrics. They put her in the front room, directly across from the nurses' station, so the staff could keep a close watch on her. Unfortunately, they got so nervous about their first respirator patient in years that they kept looking in on her. They just could not leave her alone. Finally, someone decided that the respirator was not set correctly; Jessica was breathing for herself in between the actions of the machine. (Of course, this was what you wanted. It was part of the process of weaning her from the respirator.) So the first-year resident on duty that night set the machine up to keep pace with her spontaneous respirations. Jessica had adjusted to the reduced use of the machine, and its stepped-up pace shook her out of a sound sleep. The pacing of the machine was very uncomfortable for her, and she whined and thrashed around all night. When you checked on her first thing in the morning, you found an exhausted and very unhappy young patient. A night of utterly foolish activity had probably set her recovery back by several days.

"In the incident report," Dr. French says, "explain what a pediatric respirator patient was doing outside the ICU, the only unit in the hospital approved for such patients. Tell them why you chose Jessica and explain the relative risks, benefits, and obligations that went into your decision."

When you finish this report, go to "Conclusion," at the end of this chapter.

Roger

Roger's folks have been waiting for your call. "Have they done the transplants yet?" is their first question. "It's been a rough few days for us, Doctor. But you know, allowing Roger to give of himself really has helped us to come to terms with this. Can you tell us anything about the person who will receive the heart?"

This makes it difficult for you to start. "Well," you begin, "there's a problem. We have these two boys who just fell in the lake, and we're the only hospital that could save them. They're on their way by helicopter, and we need to make room in the ICU. Roger's already dead—we think we can save the boys. We just wanted you to know why Roger won't be used for a transplant."

"Oh," comes the sinking word. "Dr. Hammill convinced us of the good Roger would bring these others. He sounded as though this new transplant program would really be able to help people. Does he know your plan? We'd like to talk with him."

You barely hang up when the nurse tells you that Dr. Hammill is on the other phone.

"You're going to do what!" is about the only repeatable part of what Dr. Oliver Hammill said. He is head of the heart transplant group and organ donation coordinator for University Hospital. His group has by now started preparing the heart transplant patient for surgery, and a physician and two technicians from the liver transplant group in another city are already in flight. The kidney, cornea, and skin groups in the hospital are well along in their preparations.

"All of these preparations are in progress," he screams. "This young boy who's going to receive the heart has been waiting for a donor for four months now. If we don't use Roger's heart, that boy is not going to make it. The television stations are coming to our press conference tomorrow. And what about my colleagues who have given up their weekend to fly here to get the liver? I've got to work with them in the future, too! If you turn off the respirator and screw things up, you'll hear from the chairman of the board himself! Mr. Stone is personally responsible for getting us this transplant program. It's going to make this hospital's reputation. I'm warning you!"

*　*　*

After considering your obligations and commitments to Roger, to his mother, to the transplant recipients, and to Dr. Hammill, if you decide not to turn off the respirator return to the list of options and choose again. If you decide to turn off the respirator anyway, continue reading this section.

*　*　*

It's a gray Tuesday morning and you have just been ordered to come to the boardroom to meet with Mr. Stone, chair of the hospital's board. As you enter the boardroom, he hands you the front page of the morning paper. The headline reads "Transplant Candidate Dies."

"I have here a report from Dr. Hammill, head of our transplant group, describing the events of this past weekend. I am outraged! We are a laughingstock. First we have to cancel the press conference, and now this! What have you done?

"I know you were thinking about saving those two boys—and about the near-drowning program with which you've been working—but that's not all that goes on here at University. We have lots of programs. While we certainly have invested in the near-drowning program, we are even more heavily invested in the transplant program. That's why we brought Dr. Hammill here, and it wasn't cheap!

"There are more lives to be saved in organ transplant than you'll ever see in this cold water drowning stuff. You should have looked at the big picture, but you were only looking out for your own program, not for University Hospital.

"But it's not just University Hospital. This has to do with society. Your decision flies in the face of good social policy. It just isn't rational.

"If you thought more lives could be saved by caring for these two drowning victims, you better be prepared to prove it. After all, Roger's heart would have saved one life and his liver another. Other organs, kidneys, corneas, et cetera, could have added greatly to the quality of other lives. As many as six people could have been helped. That doesn't add up too well against the one or two drowning victims that could possibly be saved, and you didn't even know how they'd turn out.

"Before you make another decision like this," he said as he slammed the desk, "you had better learn to count. Tell me how I can justify this mess before the board next week!"

* * *

When you write your report, explain why you chose to disconnect Roger from the respirator. Explain why your obligations and commitments to other patients outweighed those to Roger, his mother, and five transplant recipients. Do you have any obligations to the hospital and its program?

When you are finished, go to "Conclusion" at the end of this chapter.

You Turn Down the Drowning Victims

It is a month since you turned down the two boys who were victims of a boating accident. (Since the problems that arise here are the same whether you turned down one or both boys, the section is written as though you turned down both.) You have just finished a phone call with Dr. Robinson French, director of the Division of Critical Care Medicine and one of your supervisors. He was not happy. He was organizing the application for renewal of your unit's special grant for the resuscitation of near-drowning victims and was preparing the section titled "Available Beds and Other Resources."

"In our original grant application," he needlessly reminded you, "we assured the federal government that we had adequate space to handle any fore-seeable number of victims. Our ICU was underused. Now we turned away two prime candidates for our service. We trained the helicopter medics and set the whole thing up around our unit, and now we're turning people away.

"Even worse," he continued, "do you know how those kids are doing up at Lakeside? Terribly, that's how. The guys on duty in the emergency room that morning were orthopedic surgeons who didn't know beans about resuscitation. They followed the old textbook rules. As a result, the kids are still in a coma and are not likely to wake up.

"And just to cap it all off, I've heard on the grapevine that Lakeside is going to try to compete for this grant money. They're going to argue that they are closer to the scene of most boating accidents, and now they've got more space in their ICU. Although he doesn't have the physicians to support the project, the hospital administrator up there is very shrewd and aggressive.

"Give me some explanation why you turned these boys down, why we really should have this grant, and how a mess like this won't happen again. Next time we will juggle things around to take care of patients like this."

Uninviting as explaining your actions to Dr. French was, it beat out your other assignment. The boys' parents were suing the hospital. It was a novel kind of malpractice suit based on the parents' claim that because the hospital had a special grant, all near-drowning victims in its service area were actually its patients. The hospital's lawyers had called last week.

"Tell us," they said, "your reasons for turning these kids down. You had better make sure there was no other course of action. We are going to argue in court that you had an absolute obligation to every patient in the ICU. We want you to provide the medical and ethical arguments about a physician's duties and obligations to buttress our case. And we do not want to go to court with any of those scarce-resources-and-maximizing-benefits arguments. They do not go over well before a jury—they sound like doctors playing God."

Once you've written your one-page sketch, go to "Conclusion," at the end of this chapter.

Marti or Tom

These are the most medically risky patients. With great difficulty, you persuade pediatrics to take one or both. The staff is nervous about it, but you assure them that you will provide all the help you can and that you will take the patient(s) back as soon as possible. They spend an uneventful Saturday night in pediatrics, and on Sunday morning Roger's bed is available and, together with an unexpected death, there is space for their return to the ICU.

From a medical point of view, this decision works out better than any other.

Does that make it the right decision? Or was it just a matter of luck? How does the fact that this choice works out well affect your moral evaluation?

Conclusion

Congratulations! You've muddled through. You've either refused the two boys who will be vegetating at Lakeside Hospital for the indefinite future, or you've made room for one or both of them at the expense of your old friends. Did you at least use a good process for your decision? Are you satisfied using obligations, commitments, risks, and benefits as a basis for your moral decision-making?

By the way, if you do not want to face the same problem on Fourth of July weekend, you better make plans for Tom and Marti.

chapter

9

* * * * *

Marti Revisited

"Since we did so well with discussions about Tom last week," you say, "shall we try to make some plans for Marti? Let me brief Mrs. Dow who is attending our patient care conference today representing the State's Crippled Children's Agency.

"Marti, as most of you know [from reading Chapter 8, "Joey, Jessica, Roger, Tom and Marti"], is an unfortunate 14-year-old girl whose spinal cord was transected at the C2 level in an automobile accident. She is totally and permanently paralyzed from the neck down and can't even breathe for herself. Her mind is intact; she was, intellectually and athletically, one of the top students in her first-year high school class. It's very sad. She says she wants to be dead. It's been more than three months since the accident, so nothing physical is likely to change.

"If we listened only to Marti, we would give her a tranquilizer and pull the plug on her respirator immediately. She has been talking about this for at least two weeks. What do your people in psychiatry think, Dr. Walsh?"

"Marti is a very depressed young lady. Considering her condition, of course, that is not at all surprising. It's only three months since her accident. Depression is an expected and normal stage in the process of recovery. At this point it is outrageous to think of Marti's making any decision at all about her care, much less her life.

"Marti has stopped denying some of her injury and has started the painful process of learning to live with it. Our job is to help her work through this adjustment."

"How long do you think it will take her to get over her depression?" you ask.

"I don't think she will ever completely recover," replies Dr. Walsh candidly. "Compared with those born with physical handicaps, people who acquire them by injury are much less likely to adapt fully to their condition. Something has been taken away from them; they've been robbed, so to speak. They never completely get over it.

"Marti, therefore, will probably need help with recurrent depression for a long time. If, from time to time, she expresses suicidal wishes, we will take that as evidence of depression and deal with it appropriately. It would also be evidence of our failure in rehabilitation; we would just have to try harder to help her accommodate."

"Sounds like a catch 22," comments Barbara. "If you want to die, you're crazy, but if you're crazy, you aren't competent to make the decision to die."

"There may be some truth to that, Barbara," Dr. Walsh continues calmly, "but I think the responsibility of medicine is to help people live their lives and adapt to their circumstances. Many quadriplegics lead adequate, even satisfying, lives. Depression is a treatable condition and, like other illnesses, it is our job to treat it. The issue is not confined to suicide. If she is unhappy, she needs our help to adjust. She may need our help for a long time."

"As we discussed last week when we were talking about Tom's case," Professor Bradstreet grumbles, "this is a question about what is best for society, not just for Marti. Her care is going to cost society millions of dollars over her lifetime. She will never make any contribution. But, unlike Tom, we know what she wants—to die. Social utility theory would suggest that we should let her die, and we should use the money saved to educate children who will give society a return on that investment.

"Have any of you read Richard Lamm's article in the *Hastings Center Report* for March 1999? If not, you really should. Lamm was governor of Colorado and is very thoughtful about public policy and about the ethics of health care. His article talks about what he calls the need to redraw the ethics map. His criticizes our ethical discussions for looking at individual patients one at a time. We focus on 'patient rights,' on 'the patient's autonomy,' on 'our responsibility to the patient,' forgetting that individual patients are not our only responsibility. As he points out, we consistently avoid any discussion of costs and think as if the individual were our only concern. In doing so we ignore the sacrifices imposed on others. Were he here, he would point out that the hundred thousand dollars or more we will spend each year keeping Marti alive could easily provide teachers for our children in overcrowded classrooms. As he points out, 'everything we do in a budget prevents us from doing something else we also care about.' He says, 'If there is a conflict between the total social good and the good of an individual, public policy is sworn to uphold the public interest.' He goes on to point out that choices and trade-offs must be made, and writes that 'individual-centered ethics are incompatible with maximization of the social good.'

"This is one of the burdens of being a utilitarian," continues Bradstreet. "If we want to maximize happiness, sometimes it means sacrificing the good of the individual for the greater good of society. Perhaps it is easier in Marti's case because her desires coincide with society's greater good. This little group, however, is certainly not the right body to make these decisions. Unfortunately, society has not yet given any group the charge to make such socially responsible but politically very sensitive decisions in this sort of situation, but we really do need to work toward a better social policy. I'd suggest that you all read Lamm's article."

"Excuse me, but I am very uncomfortable with even raising these issues of social utility," says Mrs. Dow, angrily twisting her wheelchair back and forth at the table. "There is a group charged with making policy for these situations; that group, which I represent, is the State's Crippled Children's Service. Our policy is to do anything and everything we can to rehabilitate these children. We regard allocating our support on the basis of expected social contribution as immoral, undemocratic, and probably illegal. If you don't like our social policy, write to your state senator and representative. But you recognize that our agency has powerful organized support among the disabled citizens of this state."

"Allocation of resources is just not the issue at all," begins Sara, Marti's principal nurse. "Despite what this fellow Lamm says, our society is not based on how it spends its money, but on its respect for individuals and their decisions. That is what democracy is all about. In all the material on medical ethics I've been reading in the nursing journals, respecting the autonomy of the individual is the key to moral decision-making. I have to disagree with Dr. Walsh because he is advocating paternalism. He won't let Marti make a decision that he doesn't consider rational, healthy, and beneficial. Professor Bradstreet is paternalistic, too. His, of course, is 'Big Brother' paternalism. Don't all of us have the right to make decisions about how we will be cared for while alive, or the right to end that life if we choose?

"Marti is 14 years old, and she is fairly mature. I agree with Dr. Walsh that Marti is depressed right now and that she should not make any quick decisions. We will have to wait, perhaps even six months or more, before we see if she can adjust to her quadriplegia. But then her life should be her own decision."

Barbara, Tom's nurse, supports Sara. "In Tom's case I think we are substituting our judgment for his own—a judgment that, as an infant, he obviously cannot make. That is not the case here. I agree with Sara that this is Marti's decision."

"Well, that's not so clear to me," says Dr. Graeme, one of the senior pediatricians. "How many of you are parents? How many parents would let their 14-year-olds make decisions like this? This patient autonomy business is fine for mature adults, but we're dealing with a child from a very warm family whose parents closely supervise everything she does—the television shows she watches, the movies she goes to, the friends she has over. They are pretty careful about what she does. Now you're going to let this child make an irrevocable decision about her own death? That's crazy! Marti has a perfectly normal 14-year-old intellect and 14-year-old emotions, which is why she is utterly incapable of making this decision. I know that I'm speaking as a mother, but that experience should count for something.

"Furthermore, she has an intact and loving family. They're very committed to caring for her. We should do nothing at all to separate her from that care. It's not our business to push her toward autonomy. Her family has reasonable ideas about Marti's life. These people want to provide good, customary medicine. They are not fanatics who are turning away from standard care. The burden of proof has to rest on those who would reject standard care, and there is no way that a 14-year-old can shoulder that burden.

"I realize, of course, that the day will come when Marti will make her own decisions. But that day is many years away; it is not our concern now, or any time soon."

"I'm sorry to have to disagree with you, Dr. Graeme," Sara begins. "We start from the same point but end up very differently.

"Marti is a perfectly normal 14-year-old, and I know that life is asking a lot of her. It's all very unfair, of course, but that's how it is; it's her decision.

"My position is very simple, but let me read a passage from my medical ethics text quoting an old court decision:

> No right is held more sacred, or is more carefully guarded by the common law, than the right of every individual to the possession and control of his own person, free from all restraint or interference by others, unless by clear and unquestionable authority of law.
>
> *Union Pacific Railway Company v. Botsford (1891)*

"The right to self-determination has a basis in law, and a moral basis in personal autonomy. Lots of philosophers talk about it; it's part of our Constitution and part of our whole society.

"In many recent cases adult quadriplegics have asked to have their respirators turned off. In every case I know of, certainly in all the recent ones, courts have supported the autonomous decision of the individual. Now I have to admit that it isn't clear exactly when this applies to Marti. It's tough when teenagers have to make decisions like this. And I don't suppose anyone is ever mature enough. I know I would be terrified; I wouldn't have the guts to tell them to pull the plug on me.

"The only thing that counts is that Marti has the right to decide her own fate. It's reasonable to stall for a little bit, at least until she gets over the initial shock. But everything turns on what she decides. It's her life."

"It may be her life, but it's our respirator," puts in Bernie, the resident. "She can do anything she wants, or can get someone else to do it, but not while she's in our care. It's fine with me if we get her out of here and if she persuades somebody in a nursing home or even her parents to pull the plug for her. But while she's our patient, she gives up some of her autonomy.

"Remember the case of the woman in California who got herself admitted to a hospital and then didn't want them to feed her with a nasogastric tube? The hospital got a court to support its argument that it could determine appropriate medical care as long as the woman was its patient. I know that case got tied up in all sorts of legal complications and even their ethics committee got sued. But I think the court had it right the first time. I didn't become a doctor, spend all this time and money studying medicine, to cater to the irresponsible whims of 14-year-olds. And I'm fully aware that many people with the emotions of 14-year-olds are actually 44 or 64 years of legal age. People become our patients because they're sick and need our help. It's our job to help in every way we can, even when that involves frustrating their self-destructive urges.

"If Marti wants to control her medical care, she'll have to get out of here."

"You bastard," sputtered Barbara, "that's mean. Aren't we here to serve our patients? Aren't we all in health care to help people? If that little girl pleaded with you to do something for her, you wouldn't do it? What kind of patient service is that? None at all! Just because she's in a hospital, you impose limits on her autonomy, boundaries on what she can decide. What gives you the right to do that? Our job is to take care of patients, to put their needs first. Does she have to sign out against medical advice to get the care she needs? She didn't even come here voluntarily; the ambulance brought her."

"Hold on just a second," interrupted Dr. Graeme. "Neither of you are seeing the whole picture. I agree with Barbara and Sara that this is a question of who should decide. But how can you take a 14-year-old out of the context of her family? No 14-year-old, indeed very few of us, has the kind of individual autonomy that you two are talking about. Aren't our husbands, wives, children, and parents involved in any important decisions we make, especially life-or-death decisions?

"I also agree just a little with Bernie. We have to have a bias for treatment. Only if both Marti and her family were firm in their decision and held to it for a good period of time would I agree to take her off the respirator. Under those circumstances, I would do it; I would not pass the buck to a nursing home or anybody else. I also agree with you, Professor Bradstreet, that we as a society need to look at how we are allocating our health care resources. Perhaps we need to prioritize our public health care resources, as the state of Oregon did, but this is not the time nor is a patient care conference the place to do it."

"I'll say," put in Mrs. Dow. "My agency is paying for Marti's care since her parents' insurance ran out. I don't know about Colorado or Oregon, but policy in this state is to help disabled individuals. So long as Marti is under 18, we will provide every service she needs. The social cost decision was made elsewhere and it is certainly not in this group's hands.

"As I think about her situation, Marti might make a great poster child for our public awareness campaign. Getting involved in helping others to be aware of respirator patients among us might snap her out of her funk. She could be a teen-age Christopher Reeve. What do you think, Dr. Walsh? Might going public help her depression?"

*   *   *

Marti's case raises a number of ethical issues for you to consider.

- What do you think of Dr. Walsh's catch 22? Does a person have a right to commit suicide, or is that wish a sign of depression and therefore of emotional incompetence requiring treatment? What is the way out of this dilemma?
- Is it ethical to make cost a factor in making decisions about individuals? Does patient autonomy always come before cost? Richard Lamm argues that public policy is compassionate, not one individual at a time, but in terms of total social needs. Should we rely on democratic government, subject to pressures from constituents and the media, to determine those needs, or would it be better to rely on experts in, for example, medicine, education, and transportation?
- Would you agree with Dr. Graeme that this is far too important a decision to leave to a 14-year-old? At what age could someone make such a decision? If it is not a matter of age, what are reasonable tests for decision-making capacity when the decision will end in death?
- Is it reasonable to leave the decision solely to the individual, without involvement of family and friends? How should caregivers take account of family and significant others in making decisions, especially in the case of psychologically vulnerable patients?
- Evaluate Bernie's argument that admission to the hospital limits a patient's autonomy. Why must patients certify that they are acting "against medical advice" when they refuse to do what physicians advise?
- Would it be ethical to allow Mrs. Dow to meet with Marti to convince the girl to participate in a publicity campaign for public acceptance of the handicapped? Is this therapeutic? Is it manipulative? Should it be a matter for Marti's autonomous decision? How do the limits you might place on Marti's decision about publicity relate to the limits you might place on her ability to make medical care decisions?

Having considered these arguments, what would be your plan for Marti? On what basis would you make it, and how would you morally defend it?

chapter

10

* * * * *

Tom Revisited

Four days have passed since what is now referred to as the "Memorial Day Massacre" (presented in Chapter 8, "Joey, Jessica, Roger, Tom, and Marti"). Everyone in the hospital echoes the sentiment: never again. But it is not long until the Fourth of July, and not a minute too soon to start planning. There is no reason to think that the Memorial Day problems will not recur. Even if the Fourth was not around the corner, both Tom and Marti deserve some long-term planning.

The word is out that there are tough decisions to be made on social work rounds this morning. All the regulars, and some irregular attenders, are there. The hospital chaplain, the hospital's new biomedical ethicist, the ICU social worker, and Tom's and Marti's nurses are all there.

"Look, team," you begin, "we're not going to go through that Memorial Day hassle again. Our mistake was in not planning ahead. Joey is gone, so is Roger. Jessica is out of the ICU and should be home well before July 4th. Tom and Marti will still be around. We've got to make some plans while we have time. That's why I've asked for this meeting.

"Let's start with Tom. What should we plan for him?"

"What's to plan?" asks Bernie, the resident currently caring for Tom. "At the moment, there is nothing we can do for Tom but wait and hope. I'll grant there isn't much hope that Tom's lungs are going to develop, and we don't really know why Tom hasn't been developing mentally and socially. We should just do for Tom what we do for every other patient—provide the best medical care we can. That's our plain and simple moral obligation. That is what 2,000 years of ethical medicine is all about; I don't understand all the fuss." "Well, I can say what the fuss is about," said Professor Bradstreet, the ethicist. "The problem is really a societal one. We are just hiding behind platitudes if we talk of providing 'the best medical care.' Are we talking about the best technical care, or the best care for Tom? If we are looking at what is best for Tom, we have to look at it in the context of what is best for the family and what is best for society. We cannot look at Tom in isolation.

"Our health care delivery system is in mortal crisis. Unless we do something about its spiraling costs, the whole system will come crashing down around us. Medical intervention in Tom's case has been a health care resources disaster from the very first. Results of in-utero surgery have not been very good, as Tom's situation amply illustrates. The hospital has invested an enormous amount of its own money in Tom's care. More worthwhile expenditures have been passed over because so much money is used to support him. Now Oregon has—"

"I hate to interrupt, Professor Bradstreet," said Jim, the ICU social worker, "but I think all the cost arguments will only cloud the issues. It's not our job to worry about the costs and benefits to society, or even to the hospital. Tom is our concern. But neither do I buy Bernie's line either; we have to consider Tom's future in making our decision.

"The context of Tom's care has got to be his own and his family's situation. It is not just a technical decision, nor something for society as a whole. Tom's care, it seems to me, is primarily his mother's decision. Since it is obvious that Tom cannot make his own decisions, Rosa, his mother, has the right to make them for him. As long as her decision-making is appropriate, within medical and social limits, she is the one to decide.

"It has taken Rosa a long time to get over the optimistic stuff she was being handed by the obstetrical surgeons. During the past several months, however, she seems to be getting more realistic. She is getting discouraged, but there is no way she is ready to throw in the towel. She still hopes her son will make it. If we are thinking of letting Tom die, we'll not get Rosa to agree anytime soon."

"Well, it's not just a matter of waiting for Rosa to come around," put in Barbara, Tom's primary nurse. "Although she certainly has the right to a lot of input, we have to explain Tom's situation to her so that her views are reasonable. And the reasonableness of the decision has to be based on a careful assessment of Tom. Of course, we can keep him going as he is almost indefinitely, but is that really for his benefit? Tom is our first concern. We are concerned about Rosa and about our needs in the ICU. We should consider benefits to science—discovering how well in-utero surgery works—and to society, but these should all be secondary; Tom is our primary concern. We have to make a plan. It doesn't so much matter *who* decides; the important thing is to focus on Tom. Once we figure out what's best for him, we can figure out how to do it."

* * *

Each character in this vignette proposed an overall approach to dealing with Tom's problem.

- Bernie, the resident, proposes to stick to the duty of physicians to provide medical care independent of outside considerations.
- Professor Bradstreet proposes to look at the overall costs and benefits to society in deciding about Tom's continued treatment.
- Jim, the social worker, holds that Tom's mother has the right to make the decision.
- Barbara, Tom's nurse, wants to decide what is in Tom's best interest and to set up the decision-making situation so as to produce what is most beneficial for him.

Each of these represent different ethical approaches to decision making. Read on to see where each leads.

Bernie's Approach: Continued Medical Care

Barbara begins: "Bernie, the problem of continuing this kind of care forever is that it never ends. Will you treat aggressively when Tom develops pneumonia? Will you use whatever antibiotic it takes, including those with severe side effects and those that cost a small fortune? What about when he gets a systemic infection with one of the bad bugs that respirator patients always get? Five years from now, when Tom is no longer a cute if somewhat delayed infant, but a very retarded child, will you still be here, pushing on? No, you'll be in full-time practice somewhere else; only we nurses will be here, holding the bag. Are you going to provide us with emotional support? We spend most our time here in the ICU providing high-level technical support to critically ill kids. Most of them are successes. We can deal with the few failures knowing that we've done our best. Tom's different; he won't get better. You know that. He'll just go from problem to problem. I can't take that forever."

"Barbara's right," Jim adds. "The nurses will need support. But Rosa's going to need even more. How long will hope sustain her? How long will she keep coming in every day? Soon it will be twice a week, then even less. What will that do to her level of guilt? She's going to need a lot of support, maybe even a psychiatrist. Will the hospital pay for that? How long will the hospital continue to foot Tom's bill?

* * *

What are physicians' obligations to their patient? How are these obligations acquired? Do physicians acquire them by taking the Hippocratic oath? By virtue of an explicit promise to patients? Or in some other way? If you take the physician's duty approach, explain how these commitments mandate the treatment provided for Tom. Bernie seems to hold that this is the only factor that has any moral weight. Is a physician's duty so strong that no other factors, such as social costs or parental wishes, count?

What are Tom's rights? Does Tom have a right to this treatment because he is a human being, because he is a member of this society, or because of some explicit commitment that has been made to him? Does the fact that his survival occurred because of experimental surgery affect your commitment?

Professor Bradstreet's Argument: Calculating Social Benefit

"There's another way of looking at this," begins Professor Bradstreet. "Our medical care system is in a mess. In the past 20 years our cost of medical care has gone from taking 5 percent of the gross national product to taking about 15 percent. The recent federal changes in payment schedules and cuts in funding are attempts of government to take control. Our health care delivery system is bursting under the strain. If we don't do something to control costs and distribute those costs and care rationally, the bureaucrats will. And they don't understand the problems, only the bottom line.

"It's peculiar, but no one wants to make decisions about individuals. We don't question the $200,000 for a liver transplant or the costs of kidney dialysis and transplantation—perhaps because we might need them one day. We spend unbelievable amounts on those small premies but practically nothing to prevent prematurity. Public health measures that provide maximum benefit to large segments of the population are underfunded, but money is there for the dramatic case. Look at all the money we spend on machines for the newborn infant intensive care unit, and all the money spent on the cerebral palsy and retardation that result. Would some of that be better spent on prenatal clinics that might prevent babies from needing the intensive care? Granted, there is not enough money for everything, but shouldn't we allocate it for general social benefit, not just for individual benefit?

"Tom's case is a good example. Look at the past and future monetary expenditures, all because we thought we might be able to save one small child. The hospital could have spread the money around to help lots of kids, or it could have started a clinic down the block that would have given health care, maybe even psychological care and educational help, to hundreds of inner-city kids. Which choice provides the most benefit? The problem is, we don't like to make these decisions."

"It's very difficult to actually carry out the kind of social planning you advocate, Professor Bradstreet," Jim interrupted. "It goes against the grain of our political system. The strength of that system is its basis in individual freedom and diversity. You're talking about forcing people to do things, or preventing them from doing them. What about respect for the individual? That's been a key element in our political thinking.

"Was operating on Tom such a bad idea? Granted, it's turned out badly, but we didn't know that this would be the outcome when the decision was made. Perhaps the surgeons have learned something and the next case will do better. When they started open heart operations in the 1950s, the mortality was 80 percent, but the technique was finally perfected and now we're doing transplants. The same is true of premies today. Twenty years ago we would have cut off care at three to four pounds; now care and survival has been improved so we can usually treat any baby that weighs over one pound. We wouldn't have made that progress if we stopped intensive care in the 1950s.

"We could halt the dialysis, or whatever, to stop Tom's drain on society. But how could we assure that the funds saved went to society's benefit? In Tom's case it might be easier, since the money being spent is hospital money and we could make a deal with the hospital to turn off Tom if they promised to put the money in escrow to start the clinic next year, or something similar.

"What about all the other Toms out there across the country? Would the state legislature and the federal government ever make a deal like that? Would they ever pass a law saying no more heart transplants, or no kidney transplants for persons over 60—they're not cost effective.? Could they ever decide 'no intensive care for infants less than one and a half pounds'? That would be political suicide. Look at the mess Congress gets in every time it even attempts to talk about health care or welfare reform.

"But I have an even bigger problem. I'm not sure I trust the government to do social planning. They screw up frequently enough to be sure that they would decide on the wrong plan. They've done it before—look at welfare—then they persist with the plan just because they made a decision. I'd rather foster diversity, try many different things, just allocate the money saved to health care and let a number of different programs flourish."

* * *

Before going on, think about where you stand on the arguments about individual and social benefits. Which should have primacy? What is the moral basis for choosing one over the other? How do you weigh the rights of the individual and commitments to him against the rights of society and obligations to it? How do you value diversity and freedom of choice against uniform government policy?

If your arguments come out in favor of society, what would you do about Tom? What would that accomplish for society? What would that decision do to you and your role as a physician?

Jim and Barbara: Parental Rights or Individual Benefits

"In our society," Jim starts, "parents have the right to decide how their children are treated. This right, of course, is not absolute. We do not allow parents to abuse their children or to fail to provide education or routine medical care.

But within these boundaries, parents have tremendous latitude to decide. I've spoken to Tom's mother many times, most recently yesterday. She understands that Tom is way behind intellectually. She also understands that it's unlikely that we'll ever be able to get him off the respirator and that he won't be a candidate for a kidney transplant. She understands that he's likely to be in the ICU for a long time and that this social deprivation is playing some role in his intellectual delay.

"But when I went over this again yesterday, she caught my drift that maybe it was time to cut back on support and let Tom die. She really lashed out; she was furious. She said something to the effect that it was great when those obstetrical doctors talked her into special surgery on Tom. They said everything would be fine. It was a terrific new idea. When Tom was born prematurely, they told her that he was lucky to be in a place with all the right machines and all the smart, dedicated doctors and nurses to help. She asked what's happened. 'Are you getting tired of Tom? Are all your new ideas not working? Where have those surgeons been this past year? They did this miracle procedure but, when it didn't work, they lost interest. They left you all—and Tom and me—holding the bag.' Finally, she added bitterly, 'Now you too want to dump him.' She said that she was his mother and she didn't abandon family when things get tough. She stuck with kin. She emphasized that none of the things we are doing for Tom were heroic when we started doing them and she didn't see what made them special now.

"She also mentioned that the Medicaid worker had talked with her about the Americans with Disabilities Act. The worker had told her that Tom could not be discriminated against because he was handicapped. He was entitled to all the same medical care as anyone else. It was his right under the law. Tom was, she said, getting no more than some of the other kids in the unit. She was going to make sure that his rights were respected. At that point, she stomped out and slammed the door.

"So I think that settles it, at least for a long time. Tom's mother wants to stick with maximum therapy. From her perspective, I guess it makes a lot of sense. Of course, Father Rogers and I will work to bring her around to a more realistic perspective on Tom. But it sounds like that may take a while. It is her right to make the decision. She comes to visit all the time. If and when Tom ever gets out of here, no matter what condition he's in, she'll have to take care of him. Meanwhile, there is nothing to do but continue as we've been doing."

"I'm not convinced of that," said Barbara, Tom's principal nurse. "It will take a long time to bring Tom's mother around; you're right about that. But I don't see why that's necessary. Going back to what I said earlier, it's our responsibility to decide what's best for Tom. Once we figure out what's best, we have to sell it to whoever makes the decision.

"Now it's plain to me that we should stop supporting Tom, remove him from the respirator, and let him die. All we are doing now is causing him pain, misery, and suffering. It is fair to say that Tom has no real interest in staying alive. No reasonable person would want to live an entire life with tubes sticking out all over him. We have to act on Tom's best interests, and that means withdrawing support.

"But I don't think we should do this on our own. We should tell Tom's mother that, if she won't agree, we will go to court and temporarily remove Tom from her custody. We will get the court to appoint a guardian to make a decision in Tom's interest, and then we will withdraw support. We need to be understanding but firm with her. We must remember that Tom is our patient and that it's our moral obligation to do what's best for him."

Father Rogers intervened at this point. "I find myself in between your position and Jim's. I agree that Tom's condition is hopeless, but I also think that Tom's mother should make the decision, and I don't like the idea of going to court. I propose that we set things up so that Tom's mother comes around quickly to allowing us to disconnect Tom's support systems. I do not share Jim's willingness to let Tom suffer while we wait for Rosa to see things reasonably.

"I propose a two-pronged approach to this problem. First, psychologically, we need to relieve Rosa of any guilt she might feel. She always talks as though cutting off support is abandoning Tom. Instead of presenting it as her decision, we've got to present it as ours and just ask her to go along. It's unfair to ask her to bear that burden of guilt. How can she say she's abandoning her son?

"Second, we have to show her just how much discomfort our procedures cause Tom. We have to get her to watch when somebody's putting down a new nasogastric tube. And we have to show her how blue Tom gets when we disconnect the respirator to suction the junk out of his lungs. We have to get her to look at some of that ugly green stuff.

"We can't just let Tom's mother float along waiting for her to make up her own mind. We need to move her toward making the right decision.

"Jim, you don't think we're being paternalistic, do you? "

* * *

What are Tom's best interests? To die or to continue indefinitely in his present state? Is it possible to be objective about best interests to the point that it doesn't matter too much who decides? What would you do? Do you wish to take Jim's go-slow approach, or do you prefer Father Rogers's more paternalistic, manipulative approach? Do you think Barbara is right and that you should get a court to take Tom from his mother's custody so that his best interests will be served?

What are the ethics of persuasion and rhetoric? Is it fair to make Rosa watch Tom undergo painful procedures? Is it fair for her to make decisions about Tom's care without witnessing these procedures? What are the limits of legitimate efforts to increase Rosa's knowledge with the aim of improving the quality of the decisions she makes. Is it fair for the staff to decide in advance what is best for Tom and then work to "bring Rosa around," or is it only fair if she is included in the deliberations from the beginning? Is "fair persuasion" an oxymoron—a contradiction in terms? Should physicians stick to the plain medical facts and allow patients and families to supply all the values? Is an unbiased, completely objective presentation possible? Given the stake of physicians and other caregivers, is it even a moral ideal?

If you believe decisions should be made in Tom's interests with less consideration of who makes the decision or how, should those interests be considered narrowly or broadly? That is, should family and social interests be included, or should one consider only what is best for Tom as an individual? Reconsider Professor Bradstreet's arguments. If you look at Tom only as an individual, is Barbara right in thinking that he is better off dead? How does one know whether continued life is in a person's interests? Should this case be decided on the basis of Tom's best interest, or on choosing the right person to decide? Or should it follow Bernie's argument and continue treatment because that is what physicians do best?

If Tom's interests are not clear, does the issue come down to who has the right to decide? Is that right based on expertise or on socially accepted roles? If Tom's mother has the right to decide, is her right based on knowledge of what is best for Tom or on her role as Tom's mother? If the right to decide is based on knowledge, who has that knowledge and how does that expert decide what is best? If it is based on social roles or position, who should make the decision, and what is the moral warrant for these social roles?

You have now heard all the arguments and thought about the moral basis behind them. Recall that you are the physician directing Tom's care. What will you do about Tom? Why will you do it?

chapter

11

✻ ✻ ✻ ✻ ✻

Billy

Standard treatments of medical ethics often neglect to discuss the quality of medical care and the personal dimension of the physician–patient relationship. This chapter depicts medical practice that falls inside the boundaries of ethical medicine as they are set by principle-based ethics. All the physicians depicted in this case "play by the rules" of ethics and medicine; no one steps out of bounds. As in sports, however, playing by the rules is not the same as playing well. So decently competent and ethically acceptable medicine is not the same as good medicine.

As you read this chapter, think about what you expect from medicine. To help in this reflection, indicate the three most important qualities you want when choosing a physician:

compassionate	competent	caring
honest	paternalistic	maternal
expert	beneficent	objective

Dr. Avery's office is still in the large clapboard house set back off Main Street, the one with the big front lawn where the elm trees used to be. His children are long gone, but he still lives there with his wife of 53 years. He is the only general practitioner with an office in town. Most general physicians and all the specialists now have their offices in the building that "Doctor-Care," the managed care organization, put up next to the hospital in Center-ville, 20 miles down Route 34B. Dr. Avery took care of your mom when she was growing up, and he treated all your childhood diseases. He was the one who took out your appendix when you were six, and the one who delivered your son Billy at the county hospital. He is still your family's doctor.

Billy, now 3, is recovering from tonsillitis and a strep infection. Last week Dr. Avery came out to see him when he had a temperature of 103. He put him on penicillin, the fever was down the next day, and Billy is himself again. This is the follow-up visit.

"How's the terror?" asks Dr. Avery. "Is he back to his old mischief? What flavor ice cream did you like best, Billy?" he whispers. "Chocolate? Good. Looks like his hearing is all right. His glands have come down. It didn't used to be as easy as that. I remember when your grandmother had a strep throat and we had to quarantine her in the house for two weeks. She almost got scarlet fever. When we took your mom's tonsils out, I remember your grandfather cranking up the old ice-cream maker so everyone could have chocolate ice cream. Is it still your favorite, too?

"Margaret, I think we ought to take out Billy's tonsils. This is the second infection he's had already, and we know that too many infections can cause hearing problems. We certainly don't want that, do we. Maybe there's some time next week, and we can get it done and over with. I'll check with the hospital and let you know."

* * *

The DoctorCare Building was constructed next door to the Centerville Regional Medical Center several years ago during one of the nation's "health care crises." It was an effort by Centerville Hospital to keep physicians from moving out of the region. The hospital felt the need to compete with the growing national alliances which threatened the local physicians' livelihoods and peoples' ability to get care close to their homes. It is the heart of a physician-owned health maintenance organization (HMO) that has some of the latest medical equipment. No longer do local cardiac bypass patients have to be transferred to University Medical Center across the state. The hospital's architecture, facilities, and technical equipment, including a magnetic resonance scanner and the latest cardiac imaging devices, are state-of-the-art. Dr. Gus Helmquist is proud to be chief of the medical staff at such a place. The community has been very supportive, and it won't be long now before the health plan is profitable enough to repay the physicians' start-up loans. DoctorCare promises to exceed projected profits.

It was at lunch in the doctor's dining room that Dr. Avery's name came up.

"We've got a problem, Gus," the head of anesthesiology said. "Old Bob Avery wants to do a tonsillectomy next week."

"So what's the problem? He has privileges, doesn't he?"

"Remember when we gave everyone in the area privileges so we could get the bond issue passed? He was given privileges then, and we've barely seen him since. He admits a few patients each year with pneumonia or some chest pain. He usually has one of the cardiologists see those that seem sick, and may even ask a pediatrician if a child isn't getting better fast enough to suit him. He's a wonderful old guy, much beloved by the few patients still left in his practice, but tonsillectomies are a different matter. I don't know if he can handle them anymore. His hands may shake, and he may have forgotten how. I know he hasn't done one in the three years that I've been here. I'm worried. I have no reason to believe that he can safely do a tonsillectomy. What do you want me to do?"

"Maybe we could get that new ENT guy—you know who I mean, Wolman—to help him. That might help the new guy as well; get him known in the area. Start earning his way."

Helmquist continued, "I don't know how Avery will take it. Some of those guys are pretty possessive about their patients and their income. I don't think Avery is that type, but at his age he's probably very threatened by all you hot shots, and scared that he's going to be forced to give up the practice he loves. I'll try. We better bring this issue up at the next medical staff executive meeting. We don't have any mechanism in our staff bylaws for restricting privileges unless a physician has been brought before the disciplinary committee and found to be incompetent. And you know what that's like. I'm not saying that Avery is incompetent or anything; I just don't know. But I am concerned about someone his age who hasn't done a procedure for years. I'll talk to him.

"We need to think about this issue of who gets privileges and who doesn't. We had to make it easy when we set up this clinic, but now we can afford to be selective. Whatever we do, we have to do carefully. I've heard of a big lawsuit against a community hospital for denying privileges to some surgeon. His lawyer claimed it was done just to keep up the income of the local medical establishment."

*   *   *

"Thank you for calling," said Dr. Avery. "I don't know this Dr. Wolman, but if you think highly of him, I'd be happy to have him help me. That's the way we used to train people. And it will go faster if I have someone who doesn't shake like me to hold the retractors. How do I get hold of him? It's been a while since I've been in the operating rooms.

"See you on Tuesday."

*   *   *

Are you now concerned about Dr. Avery's competence? Is your concern based on comments by a physician who hardly knows Dr. Avery? Do you think they are just trying to keep other physicians out of the system so that they can make more money? Or is Dr. Avery the greedy one? Perhaps all are truly acting out of concern for the child and only want the best care for everyone.

Should Billy's mother be aware that these discussions are going on? Do you want to shake her faith in Avery's competence? Is it sufficient to have Dr. Wolman deal with issues of competence?

Pause for a moment and think about these issues. They are common in the everyday practice of medicine, but they are seldom identified or discussed.

*　*　*

Although the story could develop in many directions, let us assume that it continues as follows:

Dr. Wolman agrees to help with the operation, and meets Dr. Avery in the physician's dressing room at 7:30 A.M. on Tuesday. While they are putting on their operating garb, Avery tells him Billy's story.

Dr. Wolman asks, "Why are we doing this procedure? Years ago, almost everyone had their tonsils and adenoids taken out. But in recent years many studies have shown that it isn't necessary. Some even think that it may interfere with the child's immune system. The consensus in all the recent medical literature says that we should operate only if there are repeated and severe infections and hearing loss. We always treat hearing loss first with tubes in the ears, and take out tonsils and adenoids only if the hearing loss does not respond. Doctors have been criticized for doing these operations just to make money. I know that's not your reason, but since this kid's had only two ear infections, I don't think this operation is necessary. I am very uncomfortable assisting. What if something bad happened?"

*　*　*

Dr. Wolman has identified an ethical problem. Now that he has been told about current standards of medical practice, does Dr. Avery have an ethical problem? How should Wolman handle his problem? How should Avery handle his?

- Should Dr. Wolman refuse to assist at the operation?
- Should Dr. Wolman say that the operation can go on without him, or should he stay to insure that Dr. Avery does not make a tragic mistake?
- Should the operation be canceled if there is no one else available to assist Dr. Avery? Who has the responsibility to see that this happens?
- Should Dr. Avery reconsider his decision based on this information and perhaps cancel the operation or go on as planned?
- What role should Billy's mother play? At this point she still has not been informed of the discussions. Should she be? If so, who is obligated to inform her?

  Now that you have read through this scenario, return to the chart at the beginning of the chapter and reconsider the choices you made about the qualities you desire in a physician. Has this scenario led you to make any changes?

Billy

The staff's executive committee was meeting, and Dr. Avery was the first topic on the agenda. Dr. Helmquist opened the meeting by stating, "You've all heard about the incident with Dr. Avery and the tonsillectomy. Well, we dodged that bullet, and despite Dr. Wolman's absence, everything went fine. Perhaps the surgery wasn't necessary, but at least it did no harm. But we have a responsibility to the community to assure that everyone on the DoctorCare staff is competent to do whatever we authorize them to do. Bob Avery is a wonderful, senior practitioner in this community. His patients love him. But he's 82, and by his own admission is a bit shaky. There is no way he should be doing surgery. I hate to be the one to take away his privileges. Perhaps we should just put in a new rule that no physician over 65 should be operating. Then it wouldn't be directed against him."

"Wait a second," comes a voice from the other side of the room. "That is age discrimination, and it is illegal."

"Well," replies Helmquist, "Let's think about that for a while. As an alternative in this case, I could talk with Bob Avery and get him not to operate anymore, and in return we could honor him as Physician of the Year for his service to the community."

Is this the proper way to handle the issues involved and protecting the community from harm? Did they address the issue, or merely paper it over? Was the process really fair? Were the outcomes what the community would want?

How the medical community polices its own is a substantial ethical issue and one which deserves far more attention than it receives. Malpractice lawsuits are inefficient and ineffective approaches to controlling medical incompetents. Dr. Avery is not medically incompetent, even if he and Dr. Wolman disagree on when surgery should be performed. If the committee properly identified the problem, addressed it with good process, and reached a fair and just conclusion, then perhaps this is an ethical model to be emulated.

When they help physicians to maintain high standards of care, perhaps managed care has a value that has not been widely appreciated.

chapter

12

* * * * *

The Castelli Baby

Dick Bernstein was the hottest neonatal intensivist that University Hospital had produced in several years. He was completely devoted to the intensive care of very sick newborns. After completing residency there and a fellowship elsewhere, he had returned as a faculty member in neonatal medicine at University Hospital.

"It's cruel and inhumane," Rachel says. "You people must be sadists, torturing little children. Do you do it just for the challenge? Don't you ever think of those poor kids and what it must be like? You treat them like objects, not like babies!"

As Rachel's little speech ends, Bernstein thinks, "That's the last time I tell my wife about a case at the dinner table. It's been a tough day. Up all last night struggling with this newborn, finally get home for a little peace and quiet, only to endure a tirade. Damn, no one appreciates what you do. First, that soft-headed new resident asking all those ethical questions when I was busy teaching him how to save the baby's life. Then the new guy on fellowship trying to enliven rounds with questions about 'what is a person' and all this garbage about rights, duties, and other theoretical junk when he should have been teaching about things like fluids and urinary output. The residents would be hard put to save lives with all that ethical stuff.

"Getting to sleep isn't easy. It never is when you've been going 90 miles an hour for 36 hours straight. It's hard work being new to the faculty, especially when you're in charge of the intensive care nursery. Those 40 babies all depend on you. The residents don't know much, especially the new ones. You have to check everything, tell them what to do, and then watch that they do it right. This is why you've gone into medicine: to care for children and to teach. If you let the residents do something wrong, the baby dies. If you make sure they do it right, the child lives. Even the senior residents, who are supposed to know better, don't have a lot of experience and require supervision.

"The Castelli baby, last night's sleep buster, is a good example. He was born about 6 P.M. by cesarean section because of fetal distress. They called ahead of time. The mother is 32, a professional of some sort. The infant was born blue and not breathing, limp. It was a chance to show the new residents how to intubate and breathe for the baby. Even with all the attention, it was 20 minutes before the baby could breathe on his own, and he still needed assistance. Clearly, the infant was severely hypoxic [oxygen deprived].

"As expected, the baby had crisis after crisis all night long, and it was an opportunity to teach the residents and students how to deal with each one—a great teaching case. Seizures during the first few hours—they learned how to use anticonvulsants and later how to hold back fluids, anticipating the effect of the lack of oxygen on the kidneys, heart, and liver. Medication to support his blood pressure, digitalis for the heart, surfactants to help the lungs mature quickly and handle oxygen transfer. It was right out of a textbook. The students and new residents are lucky to have me to teach them and to have cases like that to learn from. It was really great teaching material and it was handled magnificently."

* * *

Morning rounds start at 7:30 with Dr. Bernstein and the team of fellows, residents, and students. Those on duty overnight bring everyone up to date on the babies in the nursery. The two-pound infant is doing well; his intracranial hemorrhage is resolving. The twins seem to be growing and should be out in three to four weeks. The baby with esophageal atresia is stable after surgery. There are only two patients that are likely to die—the new premature with massive intraventricular hemorrhage and the one with the pneumonia and lung disease.

The senior resident says, "It looks like a quiet day except for the Castelli infant admitted Monday night. He's now 36 hours old."

When the Castelli name is mentioned, Bernstein's face lights up. "He's a fascinating case with lots of pathology. A good lesson about all the problems of severe hypoxia and its effects on the nervous system. Let's discuss him in the lounge over coffee."

"Rick," Bernstein quizzes the medical student, "tell the group what you learned about seizures in the newborn from those references I gave you yesterday."

"Seizures in the newborn have many causes, but when they start in the first hours of life they are usually due to lack of oxygen to the brain. The earlier they start and the harder to control, the worse the brain damage has been and the worse the outlook. In this case, the infant was blue and limp at birth, so you knew he had been hypoxic. Seizures started in the first hours of life and didn't respond to phenobarbital or to the other anticonvulsant medications we've used, so we have good evidence that the hypoxia was severe. One article cited statistics: one-third of those infants died. Of the babies like this who survived, 80 percent were significantly retarded with cerebral palsy."

"Good job, Rick. Karen, what other problems are related to hypoxia?"

"Depending on its severity and duration, they can be multiple. You may see evidence of heart failure, and we've seen some of this in Castelli. You can use diuretics to get rid of the excess fluid, but it's a problem because the kidneys often shut down, as this baby's have. So you have to watch the fluids very carefully. Digitalis helps with the arrhythmias and strengthens the heart. They get liver failure as well and this can cause problems particularly with bilirubin. If the infant survives, most of these problems go away."

"What about the bowel, Karen?"

"These babies can also get necrotizing enterocolitis in which the bowel dies from lack of blood supply. This becomes obvious about the third to fourth day—if it occurs."

"Good. Let's talk some about acid–base problems. You've got this baby whose pH is 7.1, his CO_2 is . . ."

Teaching rounds are supposed to begin at 11 A.M. sharp, but Dr. Kendrick is rarely on time. He's one of the more casual faculty; perhaps it goes back to his days as a practicing pediatrician before he joined the faculty at University. He prides himself on being one of University's few full-time clinicians, not one of those "lab types." He talks a lot about the art of medicine. Castelli is the most complicated case and the logical one to present on teaching rounds.

The new resident presents the case. The blood gases and chemistries are neatly tallied on the board. Bernstein is very proud of how the case has been managed so far, and smiles at the crisp job of presenting the facts.

Dr. Kendrick nods. "Nice work, guys. Now, tell me about the family. What are they like? What do they think about all this? What have you told them?"

"The student spoke with the father yesterday," Bernstein replies. "He told them that the baby was very sick and might not make it, but we were doing everything possible. I haven't had time to meet them yet."

"What do they do? Does the mother work? Do they have other children? Have you told them the outlook for this child if he survives—the high chance of cerebral palsy and mental retardation? Have you asked them what they want you to do, how far you should go?"

Mary, Castelli's primary nurse, finally broke the embarrassing silence. "I spoke to Mrs. Castelli yesterday afternoon. She was pretty depressed and tearful. She's a writer for one of the big women's magazines. She's read a lot of the stories about babies like this and about the families' reactions to them—maybe she's written some. I think she understands the baby's problems. She's 32 and they've waited a long time for this child—until they had a house and were settled into their careers. Mr. Castelli is an engineer for the utility company. I don't know if Mrs. Castelli was crying for the baby or for herself. She's afraid that all their future plans are ruined."

"Thank you, Mary," says Dr. Kendrick. "At least someone in this room is concerned about more than the baby's chemistries."

"I spent 36 hours saving this kid's life!" Bernstein responds. "We've controlled the seizures, taken care of his heart failure, and managed his fluids. Look at those chemistries—he's in good shape. What more do you want us to do?"

"Have you ever thought about what you shouldn't do?"

Kendrick then turns to Rick, the medical student. "Rick, what do you think life would be like if you had a child who was profoundly retarded with cerebral palsy? A child who responded, smiled, maybe made his needs known, but who couldn't get around without braces, crutches, and your constant help? What will it be like for the Castellis? Will Mrs. Castelli be able to continue her career? Will Mr. Castelli be able to take risks, such as changing jobs? It certainly won't be the life they planned. Should they have any say in what you're doing for the baby?"

"I don't know," responds Rick. "I haven't had any experience like that. But when I talked with my girlfriend about what I've seen in the nursery this month, I'm not sure we want children. I don't know if we could handle the risk of a baby like the one you describe. But isn't our job as physicians to look out for the baby? If a couple decides to have a child, don't they also take on an obligation to care for that child if it's damaged? Isn't that one of the risks of becoming a parent?"

"That's a very important point," smiled Kendrick approvingly, "but this isn't just a tragedy for the parents. Look at it from the child's viewpoint. What would such a life be like? Would it be a life worth living?"

"Would you rather that Castelli was dead?" exclaimed Bernstein. "I'm sure that the family would rather that the baby and his problems would just go away, but that's not possible. We haven't done anything heroic or extraordinary or any of those terms that ethicists use. We've just done the standard things we do every day in this nursery. Castelli just required more of them."

"Did you have permission to do them? Did the family give informed consent?" asks Kendrick.

"We don't get informed consent for everything we do down here," Bernstein replies. "There's too much to do. We'd be spending all our time explaining and talking while the babies died. I don't think more than the general consent form we use for every baby in the nursery is required for ordinary care."

"That raises a very interesting set of questions that we should talk about at length on one of these rounds," says Kendrick. "I think you'd better get to know the Castellis and talk with them about the baby. One never knows when an infant like this is going to require something heroic as an emergency. Then you really would need their permission, an informed permission, and might not have time to obtain it."

*   *   *

The staff meeting with the Castellis that afternoon starts off well. They are very nice, intelligent people, and they obviously care about the baby. The senior resident reviews the problems to date, and they are very appreciative of the care the whole staff is giving to Chris; Christopher is the name they have chosen. They particularly mention Mary, Chris's primary nurse—their conversations with her have been reassuring. When the resident talks about the baby's outlook, things get rougher. They are very anxious about what life will be like for Chris if he is severely retarded and has cerebral palsy; an 80 percent chance of brain damage is not good odds, but there is hope. Bernstein reassures them that no one is doing anything painful or heroic, and with luck Chris will come off the respirator in a few days. It hits the fan when the senior resident brings up possible future complications: rupture of the lung, bleeding in the brain (intercranial bleeding), and the breakdown of the bowel. It is not clear which one does it, but at this point Mr. Castelli becomes adamant.

"Look," he says, "the baby has gone through enough! His chances for any kind of a reasonable life are small. You can't just torture and experiment on him for nothing. He's a human being, for God's sake! It sounds to me like you people enjoy the playing God routine. If any of those things happens and decreases his chances even further, then I think we should let the real God take over. What you're doing is sinful."

Bernstein reassures Mr. Castelli that before doing anything major, the parents' permission is required. Mary also tells the Castellis that they are welcome to see the baby any time and that the doctors will keep them informed.

*   *   *

At 1 A.M. Friday the new resident calls for help. Chris Castelli has suddenly turned sour. Bernstein rushes in from the delivery suite where he has been working on a hopelessly premature newborn to find a blue baby with a pulse of 170. A quick listen to the chest reveals no breath sounds on the left side.

"He's ruptured his lung, pneumothorax—a common problem for these infants on respirators. No time for a chest X-ray. Get me a 20-gauge needle and a large syringe."

The needle in the chest is both diagnostic and therapeutic. Once the air that had been compressing the lung was removed, Chris turns pinker and his heartbeat returns to normal.

"Good work picking that up quickly," Bernstein tells the new resident.

"Now we have to get the surgeon to put in a chest tube so the air doesn't reaccumulate. Check with the operator to see who's on call."

"Don't we have to get an operation permit for that?" asks the nurse.

"Yes, I guess we do," Bernstein mumbles. "I promised to keep the parents informed, anyway. I'll call Mr. Castelli."

Mr. Castelli's response to the request is a decided "No! I told you this afternoon that we didn't want anything heroic done and I haven't changed my mind. It's not in the baby's best interest. I didn't even give you permission to put that needle in his chest, did I?"

The effort to persuade Mr. Castelli is frustrating, and Bernstein heats up as he gets into it. "Placing a chest tube is not heroic; it's done all the time in the nursery. It doesn't require anesthesia, just a little local numbing. The tube will only be in for a few days, then the lung will heal itself. If we don't do it the air may reaccumulate and the baby will die. The outlook for mental retardation or cerebral palsy hasn't changed. They're no worse than they were this afternoon."

"Look, Mr. Castelli," Bernstein says as he plays his trump card, "if we don't do this simple operation your baby will die. The operation has to be done! Either you give permission for it, or I'll just do it as an emergency and get a court order in the morning and assume medical custody of the child. The surgeon is here now. Which way do you want it?"

Given that choice, Mr. Castelli caves in. "But this is all," he says. "You are not to do any more surgery or anything else heroic without specific written permission. I will send a certified letter to that effect in the morning!"

The chest tube is inserted uneventfully.

On rounds later that morning, Dr. Kendrick returns to the subject of the Castelli baby and confronting his junior colleague. "Dr. Bernstein, would you really have gone to court if they didn't give permission? Didn't you assault the baby by inserting the needle without their permission? Are you confident you could justify that as emergency treatment? How would you justify the placement of a chest catheter to prevent future problems if Mr. Castelli hadn't given in? Does your role as the baby's physician give you the right to do what you think best for the baby? Or is that right still the parents' prerogative?"

"Dr. Kendrick," Bernstein responds, "I'm up to my ears with all these ethical questions. I am sick and tired of being second-guessed on rounds the morning after. When you are willing to get out of your warm bed at 1 A.M. and come into the nursery and care for the sick infants and make these decisions yourself, then perhaps we can talk about ethics. You didn't treat the low pH! You didn't treat the child's kidney failure! You didn't try to stop his seizures! And you weren't here last night when he was blue and couldn't breathe. You can talk all you like, but I wasn't about to let this baby die when

I could do something simple with a needle. What's more, I wasn't about to let it happen again; that's why the chest tube was inserted.

"This is my patient, and I'm going to give him the best care I know how. I feel sorry for his parents, and I'll help them as best I can, but they are not my patients, the baby is! He comes first! All the things you are talking about—prerogatives, parent's rights and feelings—these are all secondary questions. Patient care has to come first!"

Bernstein storms out of the room.

The real zinger comes at the end of rounds when the ultrasound technician brings in the study she has just performed on Chris. There is evidence of a massive intracranial hemorrhage—something doubtlessly caused by the pneumothorax and the increased venous pressure that it produced. Now the outlook for the baby is even worse. His 20 percent chance for a normal outcome has diminished considerably.

"Well?" Dr. Kendrick asks, "What are you going to do now? I suppose you could take him off the respirator. If you offer the parents that alternative, I think they might jump at it. If you don't offer it, they may request it themselves. They're pretty sophisticated. You could go on meeting each crisis as it occurs, but there's a substantial chance that tomorrow or the next day he'll show evidence of bowel infarction; then you'll either have to let him go or fight the parents to allow an operation to remove the dead bowel. And it's too early to tell but, with the oxygen he requires, he could become blind from retrolental fibroplasia. You'd better plan ahead and avoid a recurrence of these crises."

There is a lively discussion among the staff. Some feel that the baby has suffered enough and it is time to turn off the respirator. Others feel that this should not be done because the baby is not brain dead; there are no criteria for brain death in infants, anyway. Several people feel that this is the parents' decision. Others feel that their decision would be too self-serving, and it is the physician's job to be the child's advocate. There clearly is no consensus about what to do.

*   *   *

If you were the baby's physician, what would you do now? It seems that there are several options.

- You could decide to quit, turn off the respirator, and let Chris die. It would be the quickest way out of this mess. You would, of course, have to talk with the Castellis to get their agreement, but they might be eager to agree. If you choose this option, outline the main points of the discussion you would have with them and justify your decision. Why is it so different from your discussion when you put in the chest tube last night? Then skip ahead to "Decide to Quit."

- You could continue treating Chris as you have been, handling each crisis if and when it occurs. Be aware that many of these sick prematures develop many problems. He could get pneumonia; would you treat that with antibiotics? He could get hydrocephalus [water on the brain]; would you put in a shunt, a tube to drain the fluid into the abdomen where it will be absorbed? It's not a big operation. The shunt could get infected or blocked; would you fix it? He could get bowel infarction, requiring the removal of most of his intestine and continued feeding by vein for years; would that treatment be too much? Is there a point at which you would decide that you had done enough? Where is that point? How would you determine it? If you choose this option, go to "Continue Treating Chris."
- You could decide that this ethical stuff is getting just too complicated and you need some help. If so, perhaps you should turn to the hospital's Infant Care Review Committee for consultation. If you choose this course, turn to "The Infant Care Review Committee."

Decide to Quit

The discussion with the Castellis goes well. After Dr. Kendrick presents the additional information about the intracerebral hemorrhage and its further effects on Chris's chances for a reasonable life, they readily agree that the future quality of life for Chris would be so bad that he would be better off dead. They are very appreciative of everyone's willingness to relieve his burden. Bernstein manages to keep quiet through the meeting.

When this plan is presented to the team back in the nursery, Priscilla, the assistant head nurse, has a very different idea.

"Dr. Kendrick," she says, "you can't do that, not in my nursery! You are just bending to what these yuppie parents want for themselves. There are very specific rules that you have to follow—and what you are proposing is clearly medical neglect. You cannot say that this baby is chronically and irreversibly comatose, or that your treatment is futile and what you or the parents think about quality of future life isn't pertinent. If you turn off the respirator, you'll be breaking the law."

Put yourself in Dr. Kendrick's position. Do you want to reconsider your plan in light of Priscilla's vehemence? If so, go back and choose again. If not, read "Turn Off the Respirator."

If you think you need some additional help and thought, consult with the Infant Care Review Committee. Turn to "The Infant Care Review Committee."

Turn Off the Respirator

Four days ago Dr. Kendrick turned off the respirator and declared Chris dead. Priscilla called the Child Abuse Agency, which contacted the chairman of the hospital's Infant Care Review Committee. He told them that he knew nothing about the case, but would collaborate with the Child Abuse Agency's investigation of the charge of medical neglect. The hospital's lawyer called Dr. Kendrick in and told him that, as far as he could see, the criteria of the Baby Doe regulations had not been met. There is no telling what the Child Abuse Agency would do, since this is the first solid case that has come before them. If they find that this was medical neglect, they will turn it over to the district attorney for whatever action he feels appropriate.

The press started calling from all over, ever since the local paper published the article headlined, "Physician Pulls the Plug: Child Abuse Team Investigating."

The head of the ICRC asks Dr. Kendrick for a statement justifying what happened and explaining why the case was not brought to the committee. He specifically encourages review of form 3A and response in detail to each of the items.

Now turn to "The Infant Care Review Committee."

Continue Treating Chris

It's three days later, and Castelli continues to be "a textbook case." His kidneys have not started working. Today he shows the evidence of bowel infarction and, what is more, the ultrasound shows enlargement of the ventricles within the brain. He is developing hydrocephalus from the hemorrhage. It looks like a losing battle. Further treatment seems futile.

Put yourself in Dr. Bernstein's position. Are you now ready to quit? Before doing so, turn the case over to Dr. Kendrick on the condition that he seek guidance from the Infant Care Review Committee.

Read the following account of the committee's meeting.

The Infant Care Review Committee

The secretary of the Infant Care Review Committee says that the committee would be pleased to meet with Dr. Kendrick to review the problem. She will call the committee together Monday afternoon. In the meantime, please read and fill out ICRC Form 3A.

ICRC Form 3A appears below. Fill it out completely and fill in the section labeled "Action of the Committee" with your impression of their anticipated response.

CHILDHOOD AND ADOLESCENCE

Form 3A
University Hospital—Infant Care
Review Committee

In preparation for our meetings, we have found it useful to have the petitioner be aware of the Child Abuse and Neglect Prevention and Treatment Program established by the U.S. Department of Health and Human Services. Its regulations define medical neglect. "Medical neglect means failure to respond to an infant's life-threatening condition by providing treatment that, in the treating physician's reasonable medical judgment, will be most likely to be effective in ameliorating or correcting all such conditions.
Exceptions may be made when:

1. The infant is chronically or irreversibly comatose.
2. Such treatment would merely prolong dying or not be effective in ameliorating or correcting all the infant's life-threatening conditions or otherwise be futile in terms of survival of the infant.
3. Such treatment would be virtually futile in terms of the survival of the infant and the treatment itself under such circumstances would be inhumane.

These standards are based on the regulations that implement the Child Abuse Amendments of 1984 published in the *Federal Register,* April 15, 1985, part 1340, pages 14887–88.
Please respond to these questions in writing as completely as possible.
1. State the question you are asking the committee (please be succinct).
2. Are you proposing something that could be construed as medical neglect?
3. Is the infant chronically and irreversibly comatose (Yes/No)?
4. Would the proposed treatment:
    a. "merely prolong dying"? Explain.
    b. "not be effective in ameliorating or correcting all the infant's life-threatening conditions"? Explain.
    c. "otherwise be futile in terms of survival of the infant"? Explain.
5. Would the proposed treatment be:
    a. "virtually futile in terms of survival of the infant"? Explain.
    b. "inhumane"? Explain.
6. Are there other special factors that the committee should consider? Explain.

After you have answered the questions in Form 3A, write down what you anticipate would be the response of the Committee.

The Infant Care Review Committee Meets

"Gentlemen and ladies," Dr. Orville Gross begins. "We have before us today the case of Christopher Castelli, a newborn with multiple problems. The issue is whether and when to stop treatment. First, we might approach this by reviewing Form 3A, which we have before us. If this infant meets the criteria of the published regulations, then withholding or stopping treatment will not be medical neglect.

"Doctors, is this infant 'chronically and irreversibly comatose'? You indicate that there is no way of telling in a sick infant of this age."

"Would the treatment 'merely prolong dying'? You state on the form that the infant is not dying now, but he has severe brain damage and in all likelihood would have profound mental retardation and cerebral palsy. Do you have anything to add? Has anything changed since you filled out the forms?"

"No," both doctors respond. "Nothing has changed in the past 24 hours. We anticipate that the baby is likely to have infarction of the bowel, which will show itself in the next few days. This would require major surgery to remove part of the bowel, and there might not be enough left for him to get adequate nutrition. He also has a good chance of developing hydrocephalus from his intracranial bleed and—"

"Thank you. We are dealing with the baby's current condition. Later, if you want, we can deal with the possible future problems.

"You propose to turn off the respirator. Is it 'effective in correcting or ameliorating all the infant's life-threatening conditions? Or otherwise futile in terms of survival of the infant?' Clearly not, since you state the infant currently has no life-threatening conditions. Similarly, the treatment is neither 'virtually futile nor inhumane,' is it? At this time you are only providing the ordinary care that you give to many babies in your nursery."

"Well, Dr. Kendrick responds, "it could be considered inhumane to keep a baby like this on a respirator."

"That's not the issue. The treatment has to be both virtually futile (which it is not) *and* inhumane.

"As I see it, this poor, unfortunate child does not meet the criteria of the regulations. Despite the empathy and sympathy that I am sure we all feel for the baby and the family, I don't see how we could sanction turning off the respirator.

* * *

What do you think? Is the chairman correct in stating that discontinuing the respirator at this time would be "medical neglect" as defined in the regulations? If you were a member of the committee, would you vote to allow it, or would you reject the request? Think about the position you, as a committee member, would take at this point, then continue reading.

*   *   *

"Dr. Gross, I strongly object to your absolutely literal interpretation of the regulations," begins Dr. Kendrick. "Even the Department of Health and Human Services requires many pages to explain what they think the words mean. The key words in the regulations are, I believe, 'in the opinion of a reasonable physician.' I am a 'reasonable physician' familiar with this case. I believe that this child is irreversibly comatose. Even if I'm wrong about that, I know he will never achieve more than minimal mental function. Furthermore, since the respirator will not correct *all* of his life-threatening conditions, such as the severe anoxic brain damage, the intraventricular hemorrhage, and the kidney problem, I believe that treatment is futile, or at least virtually futile, and will merely prolong dying. Turning off the respirator is the reasonable thing to do.

"I think we may have already gone too far; if not, we will soon. This is another example of what I call the NICU two-step. One step down, a second sideways. It takes almost forever to reach the final and fatal point with these infants; we just keep getting nibbled away to nothing. There's never one major crisis that we can't handle; there are always small crises that we can handle, and they keep adding up. Should we have resuscitated Castelli at birth when he showed evidence of severe hypoxia? Sure. It was easy to do, and he had a substantial chance for recovery. Should we have treated his seizures? Sure, that wasn't extraordinary and they weren't life threatening, even if they were evidence of a worse prognosis. Should we have treated his pneumothorax? Sure, we do that all the time. Untreated, it would be fatal; treated, his prognosis was unchanged. But it resulted in his intraventricular hemorrhage; we can't treat that, and his prognosis has gotten even worse. Now he has hydrocephalus. That has to be treated, since it's going to make his outlook worse and his care impossible. Treatment of the hydrocephalus brings in a whole new set of potential complications. Where do we stop? Where should we have stopped? It's all these little crises that end up as one big disaster."

"Mrs. Adams, I believe you had your hand up."

"It is not for you doctors to decide on the quality of life or on the right to life. I, and my organization, firmly believe that every human being has the right to life and that that right is God given. It is not up to you to take it away by turning off the respirator. Nor is it up to the parents. That would be a very self-serving decision, wouldn't it? It sure would be nice to get rid of this problem—go back to their world travels and fancy restaurants and then maybe have a beautiful, perfect blond girl who would wear dresses from Saks. But that's too bad. God decided otherwise and put this baby here for his purposes, just as he put you physicians here to treat disease. Maybe this infant will enjoy his life, however short it may be. Perhaps this struggle will make the parents stronger and better people. Your job as physicians is not to judge, lest you be judged, but to treat the infant as you treat so many infants in the nursery—with the best medicine and machines available and with your God-given intelligence."

"What is ethically right for Castelli, or any other infant," began Scott Armstrong, the hospital's ethicist, "is the best quality of life possible—one that will bring the infant sufficient joy and happiness. Only if the infant can't achieve a sufficient level of function should we consider death a better alternative."

"I fully realize that these Baby Doe regulations prohibit our considering the quality of life, but that is patently ridiculous. Life is about quality. We allow adults to make decisions about the quality of their own lives. They can refuse treatment if they believe that quality is insufficient. They can even commit suicide if they don't like the quality of their lives. The only difference here is that Castelli is too young to assess the quality of his current and future life and is unable to articulate his thoughts. Everyone on this committee would agree that his current life is miserable. The quality of his future life doesn't smell like a rose either. Objectively, this quality of life is so poor that it is inhumane to continue life support."

"Scott," interjects Dr. Gross, "isn't that a very subjective assessment? I'm an opera buff. Life without the Met would have a much poorer quality, perhaps not even be worth living. I'll bet that few others on the committee would attach such importance to music.

"Music may be my major source of happiness. Life without music may be sufficiently poor that I could decide to end it. I can't make that assessment for you, but most of our colleagues seem to derive sufficient happiness from other sources that they consider their lives worth living, even without the Met."

"Sure it's difficult to assess what gives other people happiness or pleasure," says Armstrong. "Different people derive pleasure from varied things. It's difficult to determine the weight given to each. For some it might be just watching the sun rise that gives pleasure. Would that be sufficient pleasure to continue living? But we would all agree that for life to be worth living there must be some pleasure, joy, and happiness and, however much there is, it must outweigh the pain."

"Scott, I agree with you. It doesn't look to me as if this Castelli baby has much happiness now," states Dr. Kendrick. "He's got all kinds of tubes and monitors, probably a headache from his hydrocephalus, and while he's in an isolette can't even derive happiness from being held like other babies. That's as poor a quality of life as I can conceive. That's just why I strongly believe we should quit."

"You may be right, Ed," states one of the other committee members, "but that's a very shortsighted approach. If you had a heart attack and were in the ICU, you might be just like Castelli. But when you recovered, you would probably come back to your old feisty self. So you can't look at quality of life only from the short term; you have to look at the future potential for happiness as well. I'll grant your argument about his current quality of life, and even the crises that may come up in the near future, but what about his potential to get better and grow up?"

"His future is grim," Kendrick replies. "He has a high probability of severe retardation and severe cerebral palsy. He is likely to require operations to remove part of his bowel and also for his hydrocephalus. He has a reasonable likelihood of poor or nonexistent vision from retrolental fibroplasia. Is that a grim enough future for you?"

"You keep using the terms 'probability' and 'likelihood,' Ed. If we're making life-and-death decisions, don't we need certainty? Death is very final. We'd better be certain that we are right."

"There are very few certainties in medicine," responds Kendrick. "You know that. The overwhelming probability is that this infant is going to be a vegetable."

"Wait just a minute," interrupts Mrs. Adams. "Let's look at his happiness. Would he have any happiness if he was as you described? Could he experience any joy and pleasure? Is it possible or probable that he would at least look up at his mother's face and smile responsively? Could he show pleasure at being held or talked to? If he was able to do even these little things, who are we to say that they wouldn't be sufficient for him? Doesn't your utilitarian approach say that we should maximize even these little pleasures?"

"Who gives you the right to say that these minimal pleasures are sufficient?" asks George Lear, who represents the Council for the Disabled. "My daughter has a very full life in her wheelchair, but I don't think that merely smiling would be sufficient for her. Why do we always make the presumption that, if we can't know decisively what a severely impaired individual would choose, that we always have to choose life? Maybe we're sentencing the individual who can't choose to 40 years of hell instead of going quickly to heaven. Isn't that equally possible?"

"The burden of proof always has to be on the side of those who would deny the right to life," rejoins Lucille Adams. "Otherwise, there would always be the potential for abuse. We would get rid of all sorts of inconvenient people by claiming that they would be happier in heaven."

"You're pretty sure of your position, aren't you, Lucille? Wouldn't you at least admit the possibility that life could be hell and death a relief? Religion has preached and people have believed for centuries in 'the better life beyond.'" Lear sits back in his chair.

"This argument isn't getting us anywhere," states Kendrick. "Even if we grant that a smile is sufficient, what about its costs? Don't utilitarians have to count those? Look at the costs to the family. This baby will ruin their lives.

Look at the cost to society—the cost of what they call 'schooling' for these kids. The cost of physical therapy, stimulation, and all those things. Don't they outweigh the minimal pleasure for the baby?"

"Suppose this family wants the baby treated. Suppose that despite the prognosis the family wants to take him home. How would you deal with the social cost arguments then?" asks Lucille, smiling. "You wouldn't, would you? You'd just go on and treat. Well, let me tell you, if this family doesn't want the baby, I can find families who do. Families who would give him good care and derive much pleasure from doing so, whether or not he smiles."

"As chairman of this committee, it's time for me to bring the meeting to a close," Dr. Gross interrupts. "Since this is an advisory committee, we don't have to vote. Let me sum up my impressions. We certainly have heard vigorous opinions from all sides. The argument that carried the most weight with me was Dr. Kendrick's statement that the key phrase in the regulations is 'a reasonable physician.' We would all agree that Dr. Kendrick is a reasonable physician; he clearly would turn off the respirator. I believe that Dr. Bernstein is also a reasonable physician, and I know that he believes treatment should be continued. Dr. Kendrick, you, Dr. Bernstein, and the parents are going to have to decide which reasonable approach to take. In the past the courts have declined to overturn a decision made by parents who have chosen one of two reasonable options. Thank you all for your thoughtful and vigorous input."

* * *

Think of yourself as a reasonable physician. What are you going to do? Whatever you are going to propose, you will have to defend your position. If you want to stop treatment, think of convincing Dr. Bernstein. If you want to continue treatment, think of facing Dr. Kendrick. In either case, you will have to explain the pros and cons of your decision.

Members of the ICRC raise many of the standard themes of medical ethics in the course of their deliberations. These themes of rights, duties, and social benefit structure the pros and cons that are usually important to people coping with ethical issues surrounding care of imperiled newborns. The final chapters of this book provide background on these approaches to ethics. You should consider this material carefully in making decisions in this and other cases.

But these may not be the only morally relevant considerations. This case presents a picture of two very different physicians. In the last decade many philosophers have worked to reinvigorate the tradition of virtue ethics, which requires us to think about the personal qualities of the physicians and others involved. If you had to decide between Dr. Kendrick and Dr. Bernstein as a physician for your child, which would you choose? Which is the more important quality in a physician: bedside manner or aggressive competence?

What do you think about Bernstein as a person and as a physician? Would you like to be his kind of physician? Do you find him arrogant, mechanical, and insensitive? Is he playing God? Does he give adequate consideration to the parents? Is he sufficiently sensitive to the child and his future problems?

What do you think about Dr. Kendrick as a person and as a physician? Would you rather have him as your doctor? Is he a better role model for future physicians or is he lazy about supervising the residents and students (where is he at 2 A.M.)? Is he more caring, sensitive, and empathetic than Dr. Bernstein? Is he as competent and medically effective? Whose critically ill patients are more likely to survive?

Many feminist thinkers have contributed to the discussion of medical ethics in the past decade. As explained in Chapter 18, feminist ethics can be considered as a special case of virtue ethics. We have presented both these physicians as males. Can you imagine Dr. Bernstein as female? If not, are you guilty of stereotypical thinking, or do you believe that women deal with patients and families in a more compassionate way? If you find it easy to think of Dr. Kendrick as a female, do you then attribute his weaknesses as well as his strengths to female physicians?

In the best of all possible worlds, all physicians would have all the good qualities and none of the weaknesses portrayed by these doctors. In the actual world, however, all of us are mixed. Think about ways of training physicians that might help integrate these two sets of personality traits thus making the choice for patients less stark. Also think about the role of character in the way you have made choices in this book's cases, and in the way you have chosen your physicians.

Finally, how much does character matter, and what are its moral dimensions? If physicians are technically competent and obey the rules of ethical medicine, does their character count? Or, finally, if the outcomes are good, is that all we should care about?

chapter

13

* * * * *

Christie

You are the chief resident in pediatrics at University Hospital. It is 9 P.M. and you are just signing out when the call comes. An obstetrician from Suburban Hospital is on the line. She has just attended the birth of a baby girl with spina bifida. The family practice residents are working with the baby now, but there is no crisis. The child did not need resuscitation in the delivery room. When can the child be transferred to University? You agree to take the child first thing in the morning and sign out for the night.

The emergency room calls at 9 A.M. to say that the ambulance from Suburban has arrived, and you tell them to send the baby up to the floor. You call the neurosurgical service, and the resident promises to come over. About ten minutes later the ambulance attendant wheels an isolette onto the floor. You sign the transfer papers and wheel the child into an examining room. The child is lying on her abdomen and appears perfectly normal. You lift her blanket and remove the sterile dressing from the cyst on her back.

The cyst is about the size of a tangerine and has some of the same color. It sits in the center of her lower back. Its surface is mottled red and yellow and flesh colored, but it seems to be intact. There is no apparent leak of spinal fluid and, therefore, no ready opening for infection. You measure the circumference of the child's head at 39 centimeters, a little above normal, so you know that there is some buildup of fluid in the head [hydrocephalus]. The neurosurgical resident joins you, and together you begin to examine the child's legs to see what damage has been done to her motor functions. From the first, it does not look good. Both feet are clubbed; that is, they are turned in so that the soles face each other. This almost certainly means that the muscles that hold the feet in line have not developed because the nerves that control them are not functioning. It also means that the child will probably have her ankles in casts for her first six months, followed by an operation or two to straighten each foot. You and the neurosurgical resident pinch the child's legs and chest. You pull her legs out and push them back. Finally, you stroke her legs and chest with an open safety pin. You are unable to get any motion in either of her legs, and she responds to the pin only from her abdomen up. This means she is paralyzed from the waist down.

Spina bifida is a result of the failure of the neural tube, the tube that is to become the spinal cord, to close completely. Closure normally happens in the sixth to eighth week of pregnancy. On the basis of your examination, you now know that the spinal cord has been injured at the T10–T12 level, the bottom level of the thoracic spine. All the nerves that leave the spinal column below that point, the nerves that branch off from the lumbar and sacral spine, are not functioning. She therefore lacks sensation in both legs and is paralyzed from the waist down. The spinal damage has also injured the nerves that control her bladder and bowel functions. She will need help in urinating and defecating. Her bladder is particularly important, since a buildup of urine in the bladder can back up into the kidneys and damage them.

Spina bifida is not an inherited disease, nor does it have a distinctive genetic pattern. Even though it occurs somewhat more frequently in certain ethnic groups and in some families, there are no exact ways of predicting its occurrence. It can be detected before birth through a series of tests that begins with a maternal blood sample. If the sample shows a high level of a protein shed by the fetus in utero (alphafetoprotein), the first test can be followed by an ultrasound and amniotic fluid sample to confirm and analyze the findings. The series of tests is expensive. If abortion is considered, the series must begin in the first trimester of pregnancy.

The neurosurgical resident says, "What a damn shame. How did this happen? Didn't this mom get any testing? Many of these cases are aborted, although some research hospitals are trying in-utero surgery that's experimental but seems to solve all the problems."

"No testing," you reply. "Mom's young and, according to the chart, only recently signed up for Medicaid."

"These kids have such a miserable life;" the neurosurgeon continued, "I hope she doesn't linger too long. That's always hard. You're surely not going to treat her."

You look at the newborn and say, "The baby is my patient. There is nothing we can do to correct the paralysis, but there is a lot we can do to minimize its effects. With special braces she will be able to walk a little, at least until her teenage years. After that, of course, she'll be stuck in a wheelchair and she will have to work hard to keep from getting pressure sores."

The neurosurgical resident comes back, "But the physical handicaps are not the half of it. With even this mild hydrocephalus, she probably has a 10 to 20 percent chance of being retarded. We'll need to install a shunt to pass the extra fluid from her brain into her abdomen, and then she may need many operations to unclog the thing when it plugs, not to mention replacing it when she outgrows it. The whole business is just more than anyone should have to take. What quality of life is that? Shunt surgery takes its toll and increases the chance of her getting meningitis. And then what would you have? A profoundly retarded child stuck lifelong in a wheelchair. No one would want to live that kind of life. Why not let nature take its course? Just leave her on the ward, give her comfort care, and wait for that cyst to spring a leak. Her spinal fluid will get infected. The infection will travel to her brain, and she will soon be dead of meningitis. It's the most humane thing to do."

"Well," you reply, now acutely conscious of the head nurse who has joined the group, "that way makes it really tough on the staff. They are not used to sitting around waiting for a baby to die, especially when there are things that could be done. Furthermore, the baby may not die, at least not any time soon. Of course, no one has really good numbers on it, but I bet that no more than 60 percent of these kids die if they get decent nursing care. Some of them don't develop meningitis, and others fight off the infection by themselves. And then you have a real disaster on your hands. You've let the hydrocephalus go, so you have a 2-year-old with an enormous head, certainly retarded, and destined for a long, slow death."

The neurosurgeon turned his head as he left the room, saying, "Well, are you going to treat the patients or are you going to treat the staff?"

But dealing with the nurse is no easier. "I'm glad to see you standing up for us," she says.

"Fine," you reply, "but how would you answer the question? Are we really doing this kid a favor to treat her? Or are we just sentencing her to a long, dull life, or even a life full of nothing but one treatment or surgery after another? Sure there are some things we could do, but the fact that we can do them doesn't mean that we should. Granted that many of these handicapped kids do very well, but some of them do very poorly, and we end up regretting ever starting on treatment."

"Well, I'm not sure how I feel about it," the nurse replies, "but you know that we could be reported for child neglect under the Baby Doe regulations for withholding medical treatment or even for discrimination against the handicapped. And I don't want a bunch of people from Child Protective Services or the Civil Rights Commission putting their noses in our business."

"I am not sure what I want to do either. Where's the father?"

"He's in the lounge. I'll get him, the social worker, and one of the other residents. We can all meet in the parents' lounge to decide. But you'll have to make the presentation to the father."

What are *you* going to say? You must decide how to present this material. You caught a glimpse of the father as the isolette was wheeled in. He has plainly been up all night. You see in the chart that he is a factory worker, so he probably does not know too much about biology, medicine, or handicapped children. You will need to start your explanations from the very beginning. How will you approach him? There are many possible approaches, and myriad gradients within each. We offer three for you to consider before you meet the father.

Approach A

Your child has a very severe handicap. While there are some things we can do, we cannot solve her basic problems. It is unfair to sentence anyone to that kind of handicapped life. It would be a lot less cruel and there would be less suffering if she died soon. If we leave her alone, there is a good chance that is just what will happen.

Approach B

Although your child is very handicapped, and although we cannot correct the basic problems, there is a lot we can do to help her lead a happy, full life. Most handicapped people do, especially if they get first-rate care from the start. Let's give her a chance. Besides, there's no guarantee that not treating her will end in a quick and painless death.

Approach C

We are going to let you, the parents, decide. We will lay out the facts and the choices as best we can. But that's all we can do. Since she is your child, you and your wife will have to decide her fate. In this case, we can live with whatever you decide.

Carefully consider which approach you will take. Before you approach the baby's father, consider the following points:

1. Whose decision is this? Is it the parents' decision? The baby's mother is recovering from cesarean section surgery at another hospital. How will you insure she is involved? Will they be making an informed decision? How will the tenor of your presentation influence their decision? Are they entitled to an additional presentation by someone with a different bias? Will the information overload of your presentation to this fatigued and overwhelmed father be improved by two presentations? Should there be more?

- Can you really live with whatever decision the parents make? How does the freedom of parents to make decisions like this impinge on the moral integrity of medical people or the social commitment to protect the weak and handicapped?

- Is this a physician or hospital staff decision? Can you make the presentation so that the family will do whatever you think proper? Should you?
- Is this a social decision? Have child abuse and neglect rules and the laws forbidding discrimination against the handicapped mandated that all these children be treated? If so, why are you seeking consent from the parents? Are you merely informing them of what you are going to do anyway?

2. Since your presentation will have a major impact on the parents' decision, is there any philosophical theory that tells you what you should say? What are the rules for fair persuasion, or is all persuasion unfair?

- Does the child have the right to treatment? If every infant has a right to treatment, does this mean they should all be treated? Does the child have the right to die?
- Which decision will provide the greatest benefit for the child? Which decision will provide the greatest benefit for the parents? For society? How would you resolve potential conflicts among these benefits?
- On the basis of further reflection, do you want to change the tenor of your presentation? Remember, you can never take back the impression your presentation makes on this father. The decision about how you present this baby's situation may be the most important decision you make in this case.

Now choose one of the three approaches to the parents and turn forward to the appropriate page. In Approach A, you tilt your presentation against treating the infant; in Approach B, you tilt your presentation toward treating the infant; in Approach C, you give as neutral a presentation as possible, presenting just the facts and leaving the decision entirely to the parents.

Approach A

"Mr. Boone, I'm the chief resident in pediatrics, and I'm in charge of handling your daughter's case. What have you been told so far about her condition?"

"Well, last night at Suburban, all they said was that the baby has a very severe problem, but only the doctors at University could tell how bad it really was and what could be done."

"And how is your wife?"

"She's okay. Pretty weepy about the baby, but she'll be fine."

"Well, Mr. Boone, I'm afraid I have some bad news for you. Your baby has spina bifida, or open spine. This is a birth defect that happens very early, as the baby's spine is forming. Your baby is paralyzed from the waist down. There is nothing that we, or anyone else, can do to reverse that. If she is intelligent enough, she can use braces to help her hobble from place to place. But she will never really walk, and before adolescence she will be confined to a wheelchair for the rest of her life.

"In addition, your baby probably has water on the brain. We call it hydrocephalus. This occurs in most spina bifida babies, and it requires a shunt to prevent the buildup of fluid within the brain that can cause her head to swell to the size of a watermelon. The shunt is a small plastic tube that goes under the skin and drains the fluid into the stomach area. Unfortunately, these tubes often get clogged or infected and need to be fixed. Yesterday I admitted a little boy for his sixth shunt operation in the past four months. Some of these children are retarded even if the shunt works, but blockage and certainly infection make the retardation even worse.

"If she is in a wheelchair and retarded, there is nothing useful she'll be able to do. If she is in a wheelchair and not retarded, it may be worse because she will understand how much of life she is missing, how different she is from other girls. Twenty percent of these children are retarded, and many have less severe intellectual problems.

"As if that isn't enough, spina bifida always causes paralysis of the bowel and bladder, so these children can't be toilet trained. They are in diapers for years, wet and smelly. It's really sad.

"We could start with a simple operation to close that cyst on her back, but that doesn't cure anything; it would just decrease her chances of getting an infection—meningitis. If we close her back, then we really should start on the shunt business, fix the feet, get braces, and plan to continue forever. If we were successful and lucky, we'd end up with a girl in a wheelchair looking out the window at her classmates jumping rope. She'd probably have few friends. What quality of life is that? I wouldn't want to live that way, and I wouldn't want that for my daughter. If we don't operate, these children often die quickly without pain or suffering. Usually they die of meningitis or hydrocephalus.

"She's your daughter and the decision is up to you and your wife, but I know what I would want if she were mine. I'd want to start over again and have a healthy child.

"Do you have any questions? I know that we haven't explained everything, but we've probably said all you can understand at one time. You'll need to talk this over with your wife. Unfortunately, we can't wait too long for a decision. If you decide to treat, the surgeons would like to get started tomorrow morning."

*   *   *

Estimate your powers of persuasion. Are you confident that these parents will follow your recommendation? If you are, or if you are unsure, turn forward to

"Ethics Committee." If you believe that the parents will want treatment any-way, turn forward to "The Three-Month Report: C."

Approach B

"Hi, Mr. Boone, sit down. I'm the chief resident in pediatrics, and I'm in charge of your daughter's care. What have you been told so far about her condition?"

"Well, last night at Suburban, all they said was that the baby had a very severe problem, but that only the doctors at University could tell how bad it was and what could be done."

"And how is your wife?"

"She's okay. Pretty weepy about the baby, but she'll be fine."

"I can understand why you're so upset. This whole business is new to you, of course, but we have a lot of experience in dealing with these problems. Your baby has spina bifida, or open spine. You may never have heard of this condition before, but it is actually one of the most common severe birth de-fects. Because the baby's spinal cord has not formed properly, the nerves that make the muscles move are not normal and the baby is paralyzed from the waist down. There isn't anything we can do to cure her paralysis, but there are lots of things we can do to help your baby. As these children grow up, they can use braces and crutches to stand and even to get from place to place. However, as your daughter becomes an adolescent, she will probably be too heavy for braces and will have to use a wheelchair. Children and adults can do very well in wheelchairs. Sometimes these children get pressure sores from sitting all the time; when they do, we treat them. Most of the children we see go to regular schools. They are able to learn normally and get along well with other children.

"In addition to paralysis, your child has started to develop water on the brain. We call this hydrocephalus. It is a common complication of spina bifida because the fluid that is produced in the brain is blocked from flowing through its normal channels down the spine. We treat this by installing a shunt, a small plastic tube, to pass the fluid from the brain to the stomach area. Although this may sound terrible, it is really a common procedure. The shunt lies under the skin and is completely invisible. We have to fix the shunts from time to time because children outgrow them or because they get blocked or infected, but serious problems are rare.

"There is another problem we should mention. Because the nerves in her spine have not developed, your child will not have normal control over bowel and bladder functions. This is not a problem during infancy, of course, be-cause all children are wearing diapers. We will check carefully to see that her urine does not back up and damage her kidneys. When she gets older, we can train her to take care of herself. Our little boys and girls manage themselves quite well and are usually clean and dry when they are in school.

"Our decision right now is about an operation on her back. We should remove the sac and close the opening so that your baby will be easier to handle and, even more important, so that she won't get an infection. As it is now, the sac could leak and meningitis, an infection of the brain, could set in. Then your baby would be in deep trouble.

"Of course, we need your permission for the operation, and you'll need to explain all this to your wife. But to give your little girl the best chance for a good life, we should go ahead as soon as possible. I know it is just my bias, but it is what I would want if it were my child. We must do this operation as soon as possible to avoid infection."

Estimate your powers of persuasion. Are you certain the father will follow your recommendation? If so, turn forward to "The Three-Month Report: B." If you are at all unsure that the parents will decide to treat, turn forward to "Ethics Committee."

Approach C

"Mr. Boone, I'm the chief resident in pediatrics. I am here to help you and your wife make a decision. What have you been told about your child's condition?"

"Well, the doctors at Suburban said that the baby had a problem, but they didn't know how bad it was or what could be done. They said that you would have to help us."

"And how is your wife?"

"She's okay. Pretty weepy about the baby, but she'll be fine."

"I'll start, then, by laying out the facts of your child's condition. Then I'll ask you to talk it over on the phone with your wife and tell me what you decide.

"Your baby has a condition called spina bifida, or open spine. It is a problem that has its origin very early in the pregnancy. There are three major problems that it produces.

"The first is paralysis. Your child is paralyzed from the waist down, and that is irreversible. While your child is still young, she will be able to get around with braces and crutches; as she grows up, she will be confined more and more to a wheelchair. People respond to handicaps like this in very different ways, and there is no way to tell how your daughter will turn out in this regard. Some become superachievers, while others just seem to fall apart.

"In addition to the paralysis, your baby has water on the brain—hydrocephalus. The brain produces fluid that flows through narrow channels in the brain and down the spinal cord. When there is a blockage in the flow, fluid builds up and puts pressure on the brain. With surgery we can shunt the fluid around the blockage and into the stomach area. In about half of the children, the shunts themselves run into problems and we have to fix them. If we have good luck with the shunt, however, there is an 80 to 90 percent chance that your child's intelligence will not be impaired by the spina bifida or its complications.

"The third major problem area is your child's bowel and bladder control. The paralysis affects not only the nerves in her legs but also those that control her bowel and bladder functions. These, too, will never be normal. We can, when she is 5 or 6, show her some ways to control herself so that she may go to a regular school and join in some of the things that other children do.

"The important decision for you and your wife is whether we should perform an operation to close the cyst on her back. This is not a very complicated operation, but it is major surgery and it is serious. If we get rid of the cyst and close her back, we will begin a series of operations to take care of her hydrocephalus and get her feet and legs ready for braces. Once we perform this first operation, her life expectancy is essentially normal.

"If, however, you decide against surgery, there is a very good chance that the cyst on her back will rupture and that her spinal fluid will become infected. The infection will travel to her brain and she may die, painlessly, of meningitis. There is a chance, somewhere between 25 and 50 percent, that either she will not develop an infection or that she will fight it off by herself. By about six weeks her back will heal spontaneously. At that time, however, hydrocephalus may have done some damage to her brain. Possibly, she will be much worse off for our having delayed treatment.

"While some people say that all of these children must be treated, there are others who disagree. I've had parents who have made both decisions. I can live with either one. I believe strongly that you and your wife are the ones who are closest to the baby, and the ones who will have to care for her.

"The decision is yours. Although we haven't been able to explain everything, we've probably told you all you could absorb in so short a time. We really can't wait too long to make a decision. We should know by first thing tomorrow if you want us to operate."

* * *

What decision do you think the parents will make? Were you neutral because you thought that was the most appropriate position to take or because you did not feel strongly?

That night the father calls you and is very confused. He asks for further advice. You refer them to the Ethics Committee. Continue reading the following section.

Ethics Committee

If there is any thought of not treating a newborn in Christie's condition, federal regulations suggest, and the policies of many hospitals demand, that the matter be brought before a hospital ethics committee. The following is an account of how such a meeting might proceed.

"Thank you very much for coming, Doctor," begins Dr. John Thorne, assistant chief of the medical staff and chairman of the Infant Care Review Committee. "I am sure you have a basic idea of what we are about, but let me remind you of a few items. Our committee was created by the hospital in response to the Child Abuse Amendment of 1984 and the 1985 regulations implementing it. The hospital has charged us with helping physicians and parents to make decisions about appropriate care for seriously afflicted newborns. We are strictly an advisory group; we're not going to make this tough decision for you. Our job is to talk this case through, making sure you see all the sides and all the angles. Also, to put the matter bluntly, we try to keep Child Protective Services and its pushy social workers out of the hospital. We don't want anyone leveling charges of medical neglect or telling us how to practice medicine.

"Let me introduce the committee members from outside the hospital. At the far end of the table is Professor Scott Armstrong of the University's philosophy department. He is a consulting ethicist with us. Opposite him is Paul McBundy, the hospital's chief counsel. On my right is Mrs. Lucille Adams, chairman of the Right to Life Society. On my left is George Lear of the Council for the Disabled.

"Let me begin by reviewing the section of the current federal regulations that define medical neglect. It reads:

> The term "withholding of medically indicated treatment" means the failure to respond to the infant's life-threatening conditions by providing treatment (including appropriate nutrition, hydration, and medication) which, in the treating physician's reasonable medical judgment, will be most likely to be effective in ameliorating or correcting all such conditions, except that the term does not include the failure to provide treatment (other than appropriate nutrition, hydration, or medication) to an infant when, in the treating physician's reasonable medical judgment, any of the following circumstances apply:
> i. The infant is chronically and irreversibly comatose;
> ii. The provision of such treatment would only prolong the dying, not be effective in ameliorating or correcting all of the infant's life-threatening conditions, or otherwise be futile in terms of the survival of the infant; or

iii. The provisions of such treatment would be virtually futile in terms of the survival of the infant and the treatment itself under such circumstances would be inhumane.

Federal Register 50 (No. 72), April 15, 1985

"I shudder every time you read their bureaucratic gobbledygook. Before going further, let's get clear on the facts of this case," interrupts McBundy. "Dr. Thorne, would you please review the facts for us medical laity?"

At the conclusion of his review of the medical situation as presented at the beginning of this case, Dr. Thorne adds, "There's also the psychosocial picture. According to the unit social worker, the parents feel that Christie might be better off without all the surgery and they aren't sure they want her treated.

"Does anyone on the committee have any questions? Mr. McBundy."

"As an attorney I hate to admit this, but I don't see any issue here. What basis is there for not treating the child? She isn't dying; she isn't comatose; while the treatment won't cure her, it certainly wouldn't be futile in relieving symptoms or be inhumane. The hospital and you doctors certainly don't want a bunch of folks from Child Protective Services, followed closely by the press, snooping around here and telling you what to do. The regulations talk about 'reasonable medical judgment.' Their guidelines for withholding treatment are clear enough, and this case doesn't fit within them."

"Well, Paul, as with all documents, it depends on how you read them," puts in Dr. Goldsmith, a senior pediatrician on the staff. "I've examined the baby; in my reasonable medical judgment I don't think that leaving her alone would be medical neglect. If she gets meningitis, she's likely to die soon. Meningitis is a natural part of this condition. She is also dying of hydrocephalus. Dr. Lorber in England published a number of impressive studies that show that these children, if untreated, die quickly. What's more, there is nothing medicine can do to correct the paralysis of the legs, bowel, and bladder or to treat any retardation. In that sense, therefore, treatment is futile. Also, since she'll be confined to a wheelchair, isolated from other kids and forced to spend long months in the hospital for orthopedic surgery and neurosurgery, treatment could well be inhumane. I think that catches all the buzzwords. You see, it isn't so clear.

"I agree with you that the key words are 'reasonable medical judgment.' But we've got two opinions here, one from a neurosurgeon and one from a pediatric consultant. Both physicians know about this case and about spina bifida. They agree about everything, even the statistics about outcome. They differ only about whether one should risk a bad outcome and the quality of a child's life with such a result. One recommends the surgery even though she recognizes the chance for a bad outcome. The other recommends against surgery although he, too, is ambivalent.

"Since reasonable medical judgments differ, no one could argue that there is a medically indicated treatment that is being withheld."

"Well," interrupts Mrs. Adams, "you doctors might be able to slip around with medical terminology and all your weasel words about 'reasonable judgment,' but there is something obvious here that is just staring you in the face. That little baby has rights. Even in the abominable Supreme Court decision granting a legal right to abortion, the Court declared that viable fetuses had a right to life. And that's what we're talking about here. A baby's life is at stake under all those mushy medical words. This is a life-or-death decision, not a nose job.

"Why don't you just face up to what you're thinking about? You want that baby dead because handicapped kids are a pain. You're just trying to let her die because she's not the kind of child you want. And none of you has the guts to say that she should be killed. 'Let nature take its course'—what nonsense when the whole point of this hospital and modern medicine is to change the natural course of a disease. You're just trying to cover up your murderous intentions.

"But there's a matter of rights here. Our society did not invest all it has in modern medicine just to save the cute and beautiful. All these children have rights, God-given rights in my view, but you can call them civil rights if you like. And they aren't just the rights of football players and pom-pom girls. Life is life—in braces, in a wheelchair, in bed, whatever. In our system, that right to life means the right to medical treatment. Depriving Christie of treatment, sentencing her to death, is a denial of her legally guaranteed rights. Not only the Baby Doe rules but the Americans with Disabilities Act are attempts to insure this little girl's treatment. These rights are moral and legal absolutes, and they must not be abridged."

"It's not that easy, Lucille," says Mr. Lear quietly. "You haven't had to raise a handicapped child. I have. That's why I'm on this committee. My daughter is 15 now; at birth she was much like Christie. She is paralyzed from the waist down. We've had to give up on braces; she's been in a wheelchair for the last three years. Thank God her shunt hasn't been a lot of trouble. She's at the top of her class at Central High. But it hasn't been easy for us, or for Mary. She's our only child. We didn't think we could afford more, financially or emotionally. My wife gave up her career so Mary would get everything she needed.

"Also, all this medical care doesn't come cheap. And a lot of the wheelchairs, equipment, and therapy are not well covered, even by the best insurance policies. I'm not complaining; for us it's been worth it.

"Mary still has her problems. When the girls at school start talking about boys, Mary is left out. She tries to stay above it all, but I know she hurts a lot inside. She has only a few real friends. Her best friend is a girl with cerebral palsy. Mary spends a lot of time with us. We're a very close family, maybe even too close. I don't know if it's the wheelchair, the fact that she sometimes soils herself and smells, or just that she's different, but people are always staring at her when we go out. Is Mary happy? I don't know. She's brave and tries hard, but it's not the same as being a normal kid.

"And Mary is one of the lucky ones. At the meetings of the parents' group, I see children who aren't as bright, who don't have schoolwork to brag about, or whose families have split up under the pressure of caring for them. Some of the children are in foster homes, and many lack financial or emotional support.

"I don't know about the medical ambiguity, Lucille, but I can see the human ambiguity. Just because Christie has the right and is entitled to treatment, and I think everyone recognizes that, doesn't mean that her parents should exercise that right for her. Just because you have the right of free speech doesn't mean that you should say something. We have to make a suggestion to these people whether or not they should play their trump card and have Christie treated. After all, adults have the right to refuse treatment they don't want. Christie, or somebody acting for her, should have the same right.

"Even if they had full support, however, I'm not sure it would be good enough for these kids. It isn't such an easy decision. Come to the parents' group sometime."

Stroking his beard, Professor Armstrong begins in his most patient tone of voice. "That's the whole problem with setting up the issue as a matter of rights. Everyone in our society likes to talk about rights, but such talk quickly degenerates into sloganeering. If we can't decide what rights people have, which rights have priority, and who decides which rights to use, all the talk about rights won't settle the moral issues. Furthermore, talking about rights immediately introduces moral absolutes that are philosophically very suspect.

"We need to think about the quality of Christie's life and the life of her family and the whole society. Thinking hard about the quality of the lives involved seems to me to be the only way to reach a good decision in the case.

"Let's look at the positive side first. Treatment brings a great increase in the chances of Christie's survival. Everyone will admit that is a benefit. She will bring some happiness and satisfaction to her parents—also a benefit. She could be of some service to society as a whole, but how much is impossible to estimate without better knowledge of her intelligence. Let's be conservative and put her down for only a small benefit to society. From everything we've heard so far, it is hard to think she will have a high quality of life. The quality may be good, perhaps adequate, but probably not high.

"The negatives are on the other side of the balance sheet. The costs to Christie are in a life of frustration, confinement, and discomfort. The cost to her parents are in their emotional well-being as parents of a handicapped child and the large monetary costs of Christie's care. Finally, the costs to society are enormous. Christie will be a constant drain on society's resources, yet the chance of her making a substantial contribution are very slight. She may lower the life quality of many other people.

"As I read the scales, therefore, the burdens of Christie's medical care are disproportionate to the benefits. The benefits are too meager to justify the enormous commitment, both on society's part and Christie's own. I know I'll be accused of being too tough for thinking this way. In fact, although it is hardheaded, it is soft-hearted. It is really trying to add to the quality of the social and emotional lives of all concerned."

"Just a moment, now, Scott. I'm not convinced your method is even as hardheaded as you pretend," begins McBundy. "As I remember my philosophy classes, the quality-of-life calculus you are proposing was criticized for being wishy-washy and arbitrary. After all, Christie could be a great singer or a brilliant computer programmer. Then the benefits to herself, her family and, most of all, to society could be enormous. Toss that on the scale and watch the balance shift. What you put on the scales is very arbitrary, and you can always fiddle with the weights to get the answer you want. As I recall, there were a lot of philosophers who argued that proportional moral reasoning could be used to justify even such obvious atrocities as slavery.

"I always found myself more attracted to the Kantian theory, which is based on the respect that every person owes to every other. Just as we all want to be respected and treated as fully human beings, so we should treat others in the same way. Christie is no less of a person because of her age, sex, or physical handicap. If Christie were not handicapped, we wouldn't be having this meeting. Our duty to her would be clear, and we would be busy about her medical care. Well, our duty is clear; respect for Christie demands that we treat her. Anything else is dereliction of our duty and rank discrimination. This is the legal duty that I mentioned earlier, and also our moral duty."

"No one here is arguing for discrimination in that sense," says Dr. Goldsmith, shifting uneasily. "But good medical practice demands that we discriminate in a technical way. Christie is different from other kids; she has a substantial handicap. As I see it, common sense dictates that we should try to do what is best for her. But what is best seems very ambiguous. None of the formulas that have been proposed—calculating the benefits, recognizing rights, or doing our duty—are wholly persuasive. And the medical experts on the case are divided as well. In light of so much diversity, I don't see how the committee can make a definitive recommendation.

"I am content that we have shared our views with Christie's physicians, and they can pass them on to the parents. I hope the people most involved can sit down and work out a decision that is best for all concerned."

"I think you're right, Saul," adds Dr. Thorne. "Now I know how Harry

Truman felt when he prayed for a one-handed economist. On the one hand, people say this, then on the other hand, that. When you see all the hands, you are more confused than when you started.

"It wouldn't make any sense to vote on this case. We're all coming at it from different angles. However, our meeting provided a good sounding board for various points of view. I think there is no choice but to refer the decision back to those most directly concerned—Christie's parents and the doctors who are working with them."

* * *

Does ethical discussion inevitably end in an impasse in which each person presents a different point of view, but no resolution is achieved? Does the fact that no resolution is achieved mean that none is possible? Is there a right answer in medical-ethical situations such as this? Are there clearly wrong answers? Perhaps agreement should be sought about which answers are wrong.

As you work through the cases in this book, you should expect to develop more understanding of the ethical theories sketched by the characters in the Ethics Committee meetings. Is there one theory with which you substantially agree? (Remember, that does not mean you feel comfortable with or in complete agreement with the character advocating the theory.) What seems to be the strength of the theory? What are its weaknesses? There is a more extensive discussion of ethical theory in the final chapters of this book.

Decide what you think should be done, and also how you think the parents will react. There are many possible combinations of parental wishes and physician response to their desires. Let us assume three possibilities:

1. The parents decline treatment and you go along with their decision.
2. You and the parents decide to treat Christie.
3. The parents decide to treat Christie and you acquiesce.

Think of what you would put in a note to the Ethics Committee explaining the disposition of Christie's case. As far as possible, justify your stance explicitly in terms of an ethical theory. How do you deal with Christie's rights, with what is best for her, with the cost of her treatment, and with the duties of physicians and her parents?

After preparing this note, turn forward to the sections indicated to see how the case develops.

If you took possibility 1, read "The Three-Month Report: A" immediately below. If you took possibility 2, go to "The Three-Month Report: B." If you took possibility 3, skip ahead to "The Three-Month Report: C."

The Three-Month Report: A

After much thought and consultation, the parents decide not to have surgery performed to close Christie's back and take her home.

Christie is now three months old, and the family has finally agreed to bring her in to see you. She is doing very well. Her back healed over, minimizing the chance of her getting meningitis. The cyst on her back is now simply an inconvenience to her parents in taking care of her. Christie's legs are still spindly and paralyzed, and nothing has been done to correct her clubbed feet.

Christie went home with her parents after a week in the hospital. She remained in the hospital only until her mother could get home and adjust. After about two weeks at home, Christie developed a slight fever and seemed dull and sluggish. In a phone conversation with the parents, you suggested that this was possibly meningitis. Considering the decision that was made, you did not want to examine the baby and document the infection. Christie recovered without medical intervention. At three months she is lively and alert. She gurgles and responds with a social smile. There is no evidence at this point that her development is delayed, although it is much too early to say much about her future intelligence.

Christie does, however, have a problem, and another decision point has been reached. The hydrocephalus noted at birth has progressed, and Christie's head is becoming noticeably large. The pressure on her brain will soon cause irreparable damage, if it hasn't already. If Christie is to die, it will now probably be from hydrocephalus, and this is a far less peaceful way to go than meningitis in infancy. In the months or years before she dies, her head will become so large and so heavy that carrying her around will be difficult. She will be completely unable to move herself. Residential institutions will not care for her in this condition. They will insist that a shunt be installed, but by that stage she will be severely retarded and probably blind.

No matter the original decision and whether you agreed with it, you are convinced that Christie has "passed the test of life." She is unlikely now to get meningitis and a slow death from hydrocephalus is medically and morally unacceptable. She is a smiling, bright, little baby. You believe that the time has come to treat her vigorously before her hydrocephalus worsens. The parents, however, are not at all convinced. Mr. Boone, with the clear agreement of his wife, does the talking.

"You know," he begins, "Christie's birth has been real upsetting to us. We felt when she was first born that we must have done something wrong. Well, Sarah, my wife, has this friend who has tried to get us into this group for a long time. Since Christie was born, a lot of the things this lady has been saying began to make sense, and now we know that it was the kind of stuff we were eating that was the cause of Christie's problems.

"Thinking about that has not made us feel very good, but our friend says that right eating can cure the very problems that bad eating made. What Christie needs is nerve food, so we've added special seaweed and raw fish to her diet. Of course, that's all that Sarah is eating so the baby is getting it in her nursing, also. We are now pretty sure that all your operations and your pills aren't going to help Christie. Even from what you've said, they're not going to heal the nerves in her back, and they're not going to give her normal intelligence either, are they?"

"No," you have to say. "Our treatment will not heal the nerves in her spine. There is no way to guarantee Christie's intelligence. It looks like she has normal intelligence now, but if we don't take the pressure off her brain, we can guarantee that she will end up very retarded. I am not complaining about Christie's diet, and I'm not saying it won't work, but I am saying that we've got to use standard medical practice to get the extra fluid off her brain and into her belly where it can be absorbed and passed off."

"Is this just one operation you're talking about?" Christie's dad continued. "And how much medicine and poison are involved?"

"If we're lucky, one operation will do it. But I wouldn't be honest if I didn't tell you that better than half the children require more than one operation, and some require several. The shunt tubing may become blocked or infected, and we would have to go in and fix it."

"And if you do all this, will Christie be normal?"

"There is no way to guarantee that Christie will have normal intelligence. But, I have to repeat: if we don't operate, we can guarantee that she will be seriously retarded."

"Well, then, doctor, we don't see how we can go along with that operation. We've thought about this a long time and, thanks to our friend, we've looked up a lot of information on the Internet. You can't guarantee that your methods will work, and we thank you for being up front about that. We think Christie has a better chance with right eating. We've seen a difference since we've started the new diet. She wasn't even smiling when we began. And now a stay in the hospital and all the poisons you'll give her, not to speak about the food, will just set her back.

"Thank you, doctor, but no. We don't think you can give what Christie needs. We'll call you if we change our minds."

Despite further efforts to convince Christie's parents to allow treatment, they continue to refuse. You must decide whether to accuse them of medical neglect and to ask the state's Department of Child Protective Services to grant the hospital temporary custody of Christie. The hospital's attorneys have assured you that there will be no trouble getting a court order in this case. You are not sure, however, how the parents will respond. They clearly love Christie very much, but the group to which they now belong condemns the use of antibiotics and other drugs as poisons. Will they still be so caring of their daughter after she has become tainted by your treatment?

* * *

Before you decide whether or not to go to court, there are some things you should consider.

1. Is this really medical neglect? Or is it just your bias that rejects non-standard medical practice? Does the family's obvious concern, love, and good intentions affect your decision?
2. Who is the best advocate for the child? You, the infants' parents, or a guardian appointed by the court?

After thinking about these questions, choose one of the following options. If you decide to get a court to order treatment, turn forward to "The Three-Year Report: W." If you decide not to force her parents to have her treated, turn forward to "The Three-Year Report: X."

The Three-Month Report: B

The parents decide to have Christie's back closed. She is now three months old and spent the first eight weeks of her life in the hospital. In this time she had a number of operations.

After her back was surgically repaired on the second day of life, focus shifted to her hydrocephalus. Her head seemed to be growing at close to a normal rate, so an operation did not seem necessary. However, at three weeks of age the head began to grow quickly, and the surgeons were asked to install a shunt. They did this without complication. Now, however, at the second checkup since her discharge, it is plain that the shunt is not working well. Christie is listless, and examining the shunt shows that it is not working properly. She will have to come into the hospital to see whether the shunt can be fixed or to have a new shunt installed.

Her bladder and kidneys also are not doing well. Studies of kidney function reveal that there is a backup of urine, and she may be sustaining kidney damage. Her persistent low fever is probably caused by a urinary tract infection. The usual antibiotics have not done the job, so cultures will have to be prepared, the bug identified, and the proper medication chosen. Further tests will determine whether surgery is needed to correct what could be a long-term kidney problem.

You hope at least that the urinary tract is the source of the infection. If, however, the fever is due to an infection associated with the shunt, the problems could be complicated and severe. They could take weeks of hospitalization to straighten out and could end by causing retardation or even death.

Now is not the time to turn back in Christie's care. The point here is to recognize that, even though you have given her the most dedicated medical care, there is no assurance that Christie will do well.

The decisions to be made at this point are primarily medical. There is no good way to predict how they will come out. The decision you and Christie's parents made at the beginning has had an unexpected but not unusual outcome. To emphasize the unpredictable character of decisions in such cases, flip a coin to see what Christie will be like at three years of age. If the coin comes up heads, turn forward to "The Three-Year Report: Y." If the coin comes up tails, turn forward to "The Three-Year Report: Z."

The Three-Month Report: C

After much thought and consultation, the parents decide to have Christie's back closed and her hydrocephalus shunted.

At three months Christie is doing extremely well. She is a bright, alert, and happy baby. She seems to be developing normally, except for the paralysis in her legs. Her parents are delighted with her, and all their family and friends are supportive. Christie left the hospital after six weeks. Her hydrocephalus is under control after her shunt at two weeks of age. Fortunately, there have been no problems so far. Checking her bladder and kidneys reveals no damage, and Christie's parents and even her grandparents have learned to use a catheter to drain her bladder. The orthopedic surgeons are getting ready to work on Christie's feet, but she seems little bothered by the casts she has been wearing.

At this point, Christie is a medical success. To find more about her outcome, flip a coin. If the coin comes up heads, turn forward to "The Three-Year Report: Z." If the coin comes up tails, turn forward to "The Three-Year Report: Y."

The Three-Year Report: W

Although there is no "final outcome" in a case of this sort, an assessment at three years of age provides a good indicator of her future prospects. As you anticipated two and a half years ago, the court ordered Christie treated, and the treatment was medically successful. Christie is a reasonably bright and alert little girl. She is on schedule, or a little ahead, in her developmental milestones. There are no signs of kidney damage. She is adjusting well to her braces. She is able to stand and is beginning to take a few steps. But Christie, her foster mother says, is a very unhappy little girl.

Christie's parents were deeply hurt by the hearing in court. The media picked up the story, and there was wide public discussion of the "crazy" parents. Christie's father seemed particularly vulnerable to the pressure and, after a few months, he disappeared, abandoning Christie and her mother. Meanwhile, the nutrition and diet group with which they had affiliated began to break apart. When Christie was about one year old, her mother had a spell of deep depression during which she threatened to harm Christie. The social worker noticed suspicious red marks on Christie's arms and legs and had the child committed to protective custody. Christie's mother has taken her back for brief periods, but she is plainly not stable enough to care for her. Christie has been in three different homes, and the present one seems to be doing a good job. Christie's foster mother is very concerned about her emotional condition, but Christie's mother is not strong enough to take her back, nor is she willing to put her up for adoption. Although Christie is a medical success, you fear she is rapidly becoming a social disaster. Would Christie now be better off if you had urged treatment from the very beginning and obtained a court order, if necessary, to do it? Christie might have been at least as well off medically, and presenting the family with little or no option might well have pulled this fragile family together. Perhaps giving her parents so much choice was unfair to Christie and not a particular service to her parents. Or was the court-ordered treatment a mistake? Would Christie be better off untreated?

To get a picture of Christie untreated, go to the following section, "The Three Year Report: X."

What went wrong? As you think back about this case, would you have made different decisions? Such reflection is often conducted in real life. At least here, if you wish, you can go back to the beginning and try again.

If not, go to "Conclusion," at the end of this chapter.

The Three-Year Report: X

Although there is no "final outcome" in a case of this sort, an assessment at three years of age provides a good indication of her future prospects. Two and a half years ago you decided not to get a court to order treatment, and Christie is now a medical and social services disaster.

The burden of taking care of Christie turned out to be overwhelming for her parents. Her father seemed particularly vulnerable to the pressure and, after a few months, he disappeared, abandoning Christie and her mother. Meanwhile, the nutrition and diet group became discouraged with Christie's lack of progress and began to accuse her mother of cheating on the recommended foods. Christie's mother became depressed and separated from the group. Christie's constantly enlarging head was noticed by the neighbors, and a child abuse complaint was filed to allow the intervention of the state's Department of Child Protective Services. The social worker placed Christie in protective custody, and, when she was one year old, a judge ordered medical treatment for her. A shunt was placed and later replaced several times. Her cerebral spinal fluid persistently clogs the shunt. Christie's mother has taken her back for brief periods, but she is plainly not stable enough to care for her. Christie has been in three different foster homes, and the present one seems to be doing a good job. How long they will be able to continue to care for this severely impaired child remains to be seen.

In Christie's case medical intervention was too late to correct her problems. Her hydrocephalus was too advanced for a shunt to be effective. Christie is profoundly retarded. She has lost her vision and, although she startles at a noise, she does not really hear sounds. Her head is the size of a small watermelon. For the immediate future, the greatest danger to Christie's life comes from the bedsores she develops on her head because she is not able to move.

Her kidneys have been damaged by the backup of urine, but her present foster home is careful about catheterizing her so the damage is not great. Christie can live for a long time in this condition, but it does not seem to be much of a life.

Are you pleased with the outcome of your decisions?

Would Christie now be better off if you had urged treatment from the very beginning and filed a child neglect complaint, if necessary, to do it? Christie would almost certainly be better off medically. Presenting the family with little or no option might well have pulled this fragile family together. Perhaps giving them so much choice was both unfair to Christie and no particular service to her parents.

In real life physicians often reflect on an outcome that turns out badly. Would you make the same decision again? If you think you should have asked for a court order at three months, turn back to "The Three-Year Report: W." Unlike real life, here you can go back and start again. After following several paths, go to "Conclusion," at the end of this chapter.

The Three-Year Report: Y

Although there is no "final outcome" in a case of this sort, an assessment at three years of age provides a good indication of her future prospects. Christie is a bright and alert little girl. She is a little above average in making her developmental milestones. She is very verbal and a little precocious. There are no signs of kidney damage and her bowel movements are well controlled by diet. She is adjusting well to her braces. She is able to stand and is beginning to take a few steps. She is clearly a medical success.

Christie's family has responded wonderfully to the challenge of her care. Their family life is, if anything, stronger because of her. They have a second child now. Their newborn son does not have spina bifida and is a distraction from the perhaps excessive attention they were paying to Christie. While there are no guarantees, the medical and social prognosis for Christie is excellent.

Are you pleased with the outcome of your decision? You should not be. Remember, the outcome was determined by the flip of a coin. If you are pleased, go to the following section to see the other possible outcome. In any event, go back through the case and examine several other options. If you have not done so, be sure to read the discussion titled "Ethics Committee." Finally, to "Conclusion," at the end of the chapter.

The Three-Year Report: Z

Although there is no "final outcome" in a case of this sort, an assessment at three years of age provides a good indication of her future prospects. Christie has not done well medically or socially.

While Christie is not a medical success, neither is she a disaster. She is behind in her developmental milestones and, although it is still too early to be sure, she is probably mildly mentally handicapped (IQ = 75). Her kidneys have sustained some damage from the backup of urine, but they are still functioning. She has had innumerable bladder infections, some even requiring hospitalization. Her feet have been surgically straightened, and she now wears full leg braces. She is able to stand with the braces, but she has not been able to maneuver them so as to walk.

The greatest obstacles to her development at this point come from her social situation. Although home life went quite well at the start, Christie's father found the pressure of caring for her more and more of a burden. When she was about one year old, he disappeared, abandoning Christie and her mother. At that time her mother became very depressed and, among other things, threatened to abuse Christie. Christie was placed in a foster home for a while and has been returned to foster care several times since. Her medical care has been irregular over the past two years. Care of Christie is a great burden for her mother and both of them seem discouraged and demoralized. It is hard to tell what to make of their future.

What went wrong? As you think back about this case, would you have made different decisions? Such reflection is often conducted in real life. At least here, if you wish, you can go back to the beginning and try again. After following several paths, including a return to the section titled "Ethics Committee," read the conclusion immediately following.

Conclusion

If your decision turned out well, should you now be congratulating yourself? How much of the outcome depended on your decision? If your decision turned out badly, should you resolve to make a different decision in future spina bifida cases? Bad results might equally be due to bad luck.

Think about the problems that the unpredictability of results raises for the morality of decisions. Is unpredictability of outcome just a technical problem that could be overcome by better decision theory, or is it a problem for any moral theory that tries to evaluate actions on the basis of their consequences? If you find that outcome is not decisive in determining the morality of actions, you might think further about moral theories based on duties, rights, outcomes, virtues, or an ethic of care. What moral theory most adequately deals with uncertainty?

Review your decision-making process at each step in this case and consider whether your decisions were morally sound. If you based your decisions on a different theory, would you have made better decisions? Would they have come out differently? Try going through the case basing your decision on utilitarian models, on rights, or on obligations. Has one theory now emerged as the most plausible? Do they lead to different outcomes?

Comment

This presentation of Christie does not do justice to the many alternative decisions possible in a case of spina bifida. If the parents decided not to treat, you could have obtained a court order for treatment and had Christie adopted by a caring family. If, on the other hand, you agreed with their decision, the child might have died and the family might then have had other, normal children. If you and the parents had been enthusiastic about treatment, the infant might have done well, or badly, or somewhere in between. However, at the time of the initial decision, neither you, the family, the committee, nor the courts can accurately predict the outcome for any of the involved parties.

PART
IV

CONCEPTION AND GESTATION

chapter

14

* * * * *

The Harrisons' Plans

The Harrisons were getting more excited with each passing day. Their baby was due in two months. The room was ready, piles of blue baby clothes were stacked in the crib, and Judy's folks had sent word that they were ready to start a college fund for their grandson or granddaughter.

While all babies are special, this one was a little extra-special, for Judy would not be giving birth herself. Judy and Frank had been married almost 15 years; they had met when Judy was part of the team that audited the bank where Frank worked. Judy was then beginning her career as an accountant; Frank was an assistant manager. Both had prospered in their respective careers. Frank was now a vice president well on his way to senior vice president. Having served her time with a major accounting firm and then worked for a small college for several years, Judy had started her own firm. Frank's stable work had enabled Judy to take this major risk, and they had decided that starting a family was too much for them—until now. Judy had brought several younger accountants into partnership with her, and she felt she could now move away from the pressure and stress of her career.

Judy knew that she had a medical problem even before she and Frank decided to begin their family. She had a long history of endometriosis that had required extensive hormone treatment and two surgeries. They tried for about a year after she went off the pill, but pregnancy just wasn't happening. A fertility work-up only confirmed what Judy had known; the endometriosis was making pregnancy virtually impossible. In vitro fertilization was not likely to help. They looked into adoption, but the number of healthy babies available from reputable agencies was so small that their chances of getting one within the next few years seemed remote. There were some lawyers in their city who had arranged surrogate mother contracts; indeed, one of the partners in a friend's law firm had participated in a locally famous lawsuit in which the surrogate had decided to keep the baby. That had furnished plenty of cocktail party discussions at the time, so both Frank and Judy were familiar with the issues involved. Still, they felt that a surrogate was the most promising path to follow.

When Frank and Judy contacted the law firm, they were invited for a conference with one of the partners. Having been burned in the previous law suit, Mr. Devoe was very precise. He wanted everything out on the table and fully understood ahead of time. He carefully explained that the state supreme court had ruled that surrogacy contracts were not enforceable. If a woman bore a child for them and decided not to give up her parental rights after the baby's birth, the courts would not make her give them the baby. If they could prove that the woman was an incompetent parent, they might be able to argue that the best interests of the child required that they have custody. But this strategy was tricky because they did not want the genes of an incompetent person passed on to their child. The lawyer said, however, that his firm had drawn up a special "nonbinding agreement" for use in situations like this. The firm also had recruited a small group of women who had agreed to participate in surrogate motherhood. The practice was not in any way illegal. The only restriction was that the nonbinding agreement was not enforceable by the courts and all parties had to be clear about that. The law firm earned its fee by recruiting and screening potential mothers and handling all negotiations between the couples who wished to have children and the surrogate mothers. The women received between $10,000 and $20,000 for being a surrogate, plus all medical expenses, and the law firm added 20 percent to those fees. The firm also handled the legal requirements for adoption after the baby's birth.

After much soul searching, Frank and Judy decided that this was the way to go. If they were to have a child, at least one-half of the genes would be theirs—at least Frank's. Perhaps the child would inherit Frank's gray eyes, intelligence, and easygoing personality. They looked through a dossier the law firm maintained with photos and background on the women who were willing to be surrogate mothers. After almost a week of evaluating the pros and cons of each, they picked Bea. She was 29 years old, married for ten years, and the mother of three children. She had dropped out of college with her first pregnancy. The dossier explained that her husband drove a long-distance moving truck and was away from home for weeks at a time. The youngest of their three children was about to start school; they could not afford more children of their own. Bea had enjoyed her pregnancies and "loved bringing a new life into the world." Since Bea had no job skills, this seemed like a good way for her to supplement her family's income. She was a healthy woman with a history of three uneventful pregnancies. She had not yet participated in the surrogate program.

The couples agreed not to meet, but the law firm's negotiations with Bea went very smoothly. She had been in the firm's book for six months and was anxious to begin. Bea, her husband John, Frank, and Judy all signed the agreement.

The Harrisons' Plans

Frank and Judy agreed to pay $5,000 at the beginning, $1,000 per month of the pregnancy, and $5,000 at delivery, plus the medical expenses. It was higher than the usual rate, but they didn't want to haggle over the price of their first-born. They could afford it. Frank arranged for sperm donation. Bea was pregnant on the first attempt. Everything was off to a smooth start.

* * *

Wasn't that easy? Just another simple commercial transaction. Don't you wish that all business transactions would go so smoothly? One party cheerfully sells what another wants for a mutually agreed-upon price. Pause here to think of some of the issues that surrogate motherhood itself raises:

- Is surrogacy immoral because the surrogate becomes a kind of prostitute, selling her body or renting her womb for a price? Is prostitution morally acceptable? (It is legal in some states and many countries.) Is it a legitimate way for people to earn money? Does surrogate motherhood enslave women to a patriarchal system or liberate women to make their own choices?
- Is surrogacy morally praiseworthy as an act of generosity, giving something of oneself to another who is in need? How does being a surrogate mother differ morally from giving up a child for adoption?
- What view should the law take of the practice of surrogacy? Should it make the practice illegal? Should it refuse to enforce surrogacy contracts (as our case supposes), putting them outside the law? Or should it enforce these contracts as it would any other business arrangement? If the law treats surrogacy as different from other contracts, is it using the law to enforce morality? Is this always objectionable?
- Will surrogate motherhood have any traumatic effect on children who are born this way? Will its impact be different from other forms of adoption?
- Should surrogacy agreements include a clause about terminating the pregnancy? If the fetus were found to have a major birth defect, could it be aborted? Who would decide in this case, the Harrisons or Bea?
- Is it morally acceptable for a woman to ask for a child back after she has released the baby for adoption? If you were a state legislator, would you recommend a mandatory waiting or "cooling-off" period between birth and adoption?

Several of these questions raise issues of law as well as morality. As observed in Chapters 18 and 19, many issues in medical ethics intertwine law and morality, public and private issues. When state legislatures in the United States decide to make surrogacy contracts unenforceable, they are making such arrangements private, not public. They are moving them outside the scope of the law. These laws are based on a view about areas of life in which the law should not intervene, and are structured by an ethical view of the legitimate scope of public regulation. Much of American public life is devoted to arguing the legitimate scope of public regulation.

* * *

Through the first seven months, everything about the pregnancy was extremely smooth. Ultrasound scans were done at the end of the first and second trimester. They showed a normally developing male fetus. Alphafetoprotein testing did not flag any problems. That is why the Harrisons were so unprepared.

The lawyer who had handled all the negotiations for the Harrisons called early one morning. Bea had driven herself to the emergency room that morning, apparently in premature labor. The resident on duty thought he detected fetal distress, and called in Bea's obstetrician. The obstetrician confirmed the early signs of fetal distress and recommended a cesarean section (C-section). If the changes in the fetal heart rate became more pronounced, he said, the cesarean section would become an emergency. But for now there was some time to discuss it. This was fortunate, the lawyer reported, since Bea was adamantly refusing the surgery.

* * *

Put yourself in Frank and Judy's position. They are thinking that *their* baby is at risk. They have looked at the ultrasound scans and intently followed the progress of Bea's pregnancy. While distancing themselves in some way from Bea, they have felt a deep personal involvement. Moreover, they have been making regular payments to the obstetrician to cover the costs of Bea's prenatal care. Their lawyer has been paid and he has been making payments to Bea under the terms of the agreement. Whose baby is it now?

* * *

After an agonizing personal discussion, Frank and Judy decide to go to the hospital. They call the lawyer who agrees to meet them there. Bea had signed an agreement to make her medical records available to the Harrisons when she began the pregnancy. The obstetrician who has cared for Bea from the beginning takes this as authorization to fully discuss Bea's situation with the Harrisons. Mr. Devoe and the Harrisons gather in the conference room and the obstetrician explains: "Since the start of this pregnancy is so well documented, we know that the fetus is 32 weeks gestation. That's premature but shouldn't pose any serious problems. We've given Bea some steroids to accelerate development of the fetus's lungs, so there should not be a problem with lung development after birth. Bea is now in the second stage of labor, and the problem is a classic—breech presentation. It is as though the fetus is sitting down and trying to come through the birth canal butt first. We can try to manipulate these babies, actually rotate the baby inside the womb, but it is a time-consuming and risky strategy. Some of the older obstetricians got really good at it. But, to be honest with you, I've only seen it done once or twice. I've never tried it myself. It is not the breech presentation that is causing the problem, however. When children come out breech, sometimes the umbilical cord falls down and gets trapped between the baby and the pelvis. This means that the blood supply to the baby can be interrupted. This has already happened once to Bea. We've pushed the cord back in, and things look fine for now. However, if it slips again, we have to be ready to do an emergency C-section, otherwise the baby may develop severe brain damage from lack of oxygen. Cesarean sections are the standard of care in these cases. Anything else risks the legal liability that accompanies a bad outcome.

"Our problem is that Bea is adamant about not having a C-section. She says she has always been afraid of surgery. Her three easy, normal deliveries gave her the confidence to go ahead with this pregnancy. But she's afraid that once she has a C-section she'll need them for any future deliveries. And she doesn't want to close the door on the possibility of having another child of her own by a normal delivery, or of having more surrogate children either.

"The overwhelming risk here is to the fetus. From a technical point of view, Bea is going to be roughed up a little no matter which course we take. But she'll come out fine; her risks don't change whether we do cesarean or vaginal delivery. It's the fetus that bears the brunt of the risk. The risk of death is small, but brain damage due to lack of oxygen becomes highly probable. With the current legal climate most of us would do the section now and avoid any risk. That's one of the reasons why such a huge percentage of the deliveries in this country are by C-section. It is probably safe to wait a little while since we are carefully monitoring the baby. But if things take a turn for the worse, we'll have to move fast.

"I'm not sure what to do about Bea, however. She will not agree to the procedure, and she is my patient. Believe me, I have spent the last two hours trying to persuade her. From the way her labor is progressing, I'd say we have about two more hours."

The Harrison's lawyer is ambivalent on the subject of getting a court order. He had looked at the precedents while preparing for the trial his firm had been involved in. "Some judges go one way, some another," was the best he could tell the Harrisons. But he added: "This kind of case gets a lot of publicity. It won't be pleasant. It can destroy your privacy, generate crank letters from all over the country, plant TV reporters outside your front door, even ruin your business or career. It's the last thing in the world you want."

"Next to a dead or brain-damaged child," snapped Judy.

* * *

Many questions arise at this point in the case.

- What are fair methods of persuasion? Should the obstetrician just present the facts and let them do the persuading? Is it fair to appeal to whatever maternal feelings Bea may have, even though she is not the woman who will mother this child to adulthood? Is it fair to appeal to the money she has received for her pregnancy services? Should Frank and Judy confront Bea, whom they have never met before, to persuade her to undergo the surgery? If so, what approach should they take? What would be both rhetorically effective and morally acceptable?
- If Bea has freely undertaken this pregnancy, is she free to carry it out any way she believes appropriate? It is, after all, her body. Is it her right to refuse surgery for any reason whatsoever?
- Should the courts become involved? The fetus that physicians talk about is, in this case, a completely viable, potentially normal, healthy baby. Do the government and child protective services have a stake in protecting this baby's access to a nonhandicapped life? If the child is handicapped by the birth process, he will be far more expensive to raise both for parents and the state. Special education is very expensive. Does this financial consideration or its role as the "parent of last resort" give the state a stake in the decision sufficient for the courts to intervene?
- What will happen to the baby if he is born with moderate or severe brain damage? Since the agreement did not specify that the Harrisons had to take "damaged goods," are they required to accept the baby? The agreement did not guarantee a perfect baby, either.
- This case can be viewed as a conflict of rights: of Bea's right to control her body, the baby's right to an unimpaired life, and Frank and Judy's right to parent a healthy child they have agreed to raise. One of the standard objections to rights-based medical ethics is its apparent inability to move beyond impasses such as this one. Can you see a clearly stronger right that breaks this impasse and directs a decision?
- Does an ethic of virtue shed any light on the situation? Does Bea need to face surgery with courage? Have these characters acted virtuously in getting into their present situation? Is there a virtuous way out of it?
- Is there a single clear decision-maker, a single person or entity (such as the state) whose decision would be accepted as fair?

Time is of the essence. Put yourself in Frank and Judy's place. What should you do?

chapter
15
* * * * *

The Smyth Saga

"Robert? Are you asleep yet, dear? The dance tonight for all those poor children. . . . I really think I'd like to be more involved with a charity like that. Maybe with my advertising background I could be of some help."

"Hmm?"

"I don't know what I'd do if I had to cope with a handicapped child. Maybe we shouldn't have children. Maybe we're too old, too settled in our professional lives. Do you think so? But then I think of my niece, Amy—she's so precious, so cute. It would be fun. I'd even cut back my work at the agency for one like that. I've been thinking about going to that Genetics Counseling Center and seeing what they have to say. Would you come with me?"

"Darling, we're not getting married until September. Do we have to make a decision tonight?"

"Of course not. Good night, sweet."

* * *

"You're 32, Virginia, and in good health. Is that correct? Any problems in your family? No? Your mother is now 57 and in good health. Your father is 60 and well. One sister, 27, and she has just one daughter. I see you have no children by your first marriage? Okay. Well, Virginia, was there a specific problem you had in mind? Your family history looks pretty clean. You are getting a bit older, but not to the age where Downs syndrome becomes a significant risk. There are some standard tests your obstetrician will run early in your pregnancy—when and if you get pregnant—that will screen for many of the common abnormalities. Also, there are now some tests for genes that predispose to various conditions, but we don't know that the baby will actually develop the disease. Take colon cancer. We know the genes that indicate a greater-than-average risk of getting that cancer, but it only means that, as the people with increased risk get older, they need to be carefully observed, not that they will get it. There's nothing we can do about these predispositions in utero. A family history tells us what to look for since genetic fishing expeditions aren't very productive. Even the most sophisticated tests don't guarantee a healthy baby.

"On the basis of the history you've given me, however, your risks appear very small—no greater than anyone else's. Are there any special problems on your fiancé's side of the family? Why don't you check? If there aren't, I don't think you have much to worry about. Why don't you make another appointment if you have special concerns or when you're pregnant, but do it early in the pregnancy."

*   *   *

"This is one of my favorite restaurants, Robert. I think I'll have the veal again. Thank goodness for credit cards. I went to the Genetics Counseling Center today and the counselor told me not to worry, that 32 wasn't too old and that there was nothing in my family to worry about. She said to ask about your side. Do you have anything hidden I don't know about, dear?"

"Only my Uncle Charles, with two heads. Or is it two personalities? Good Puritan stock. Dad has only the one brother, and his kids are fine, and you know my two children. I guess that's it. I'll ask my father if there's anything if you want me to. Now that I think about it, I believe Dad had a sister who died; I'll ask him."

*   *   *

"Look, Virginia, lay off. It seems to be all you've got on your mind these past two weeks. I'll tell you one more time. All Dad said was that his sister got rheumatic fever or chorea or something in her 30s; it got worse and drove her crazy. She ended up in a mental institution. That's it. Now you've got Aunt Libby, Charles's wife, all stirred up about his Parkinson's disease. What's this about Huntington's disease, anyway? What is it, and what's it got to do with us?"

"Robert, don't get so upset. This is important, dear. Just take a look at this pamphlet about Huntington's disease that I picked up today at the center. Could this be what your aunt had? I've underlined the important parts. It's very frightening—maybe for you, and even for our children."

Huntington's Disease—The Terrible Killer

Huntington's disease is a progressive degenerative disease characterized by changes in personality, and the gradual onset of a movement disorder leading to progressive intellectual deterioration and death. While occasionally taking a different and more severe form in childhood, it usually begins in the third, fourth, or fifth decades of life with subtle alterations in movements—sometimes thought to be tics. These progress over several years. The movements may precede the intellectual deterioration or follow subtle intellectual and emotional changes. The movements and intellectual problems gradually become so severe that the individuals are unable to care for themselves. They often spend their last years in a nursing home or institution.

Huntington's disease is an autosomal dominant trait. Each child of an affected parent has a 50 percent chance of having the disease, even if the disease is not visible in the parent. Every person who carries the gene will pass it, on average, to half of their children. Thus, many people from families that carry the gene elect not to have children.

There is no known therapy. With your past support we have made great strides in genetic testing for this disorder, and individuals can now have testing to find if they are afflicted with the disease. Research now shows promise of finding a treatment and, perhaps some day, even a cure.

The Huntington's Disease Committee

"That's grim," states Robert. "Terrific bedtime reading, but what's it got to do with us?"

"Well, yesterday I was talking with your Aunt Libby. Charles's doctor had been asking them about diseases in the family. It seems that Charles's Parkinsonism isn't behaving the way it's supposed to and the name Huntington's disease came up. They were asking how his father died, his mother, and then this sister. Her death seemed to intrigue them. Charles said Henry, your father, has all that information since he handled the estate. You know, I don't believe Charles's mind is as sharp as it used to be."

*   *   *

Mr. Smyth picks up the phone. "Yes, Dr. Gunderson," he responds. "You're my brother Charles's doctor aren't you? I've been expecting your call. I know quite a bit about Huntington's disease. That is how my sister died. She was about 50 when she passed away. An autopsy was done; I have the report. . . . No, I haven't told anyone in the family. There didn't seem to be much point, and I don't think that you should tell the others either. I want to emphasize that this is a confidential conversation between you and me. Let me explain.

"When Mary died, Charles already had two young children and wasn't planning to have more. Robert was 10, and my wife and I had already decided not to have more children. Charles was always a hypochondriac—rushing off to doctors with each little ache or pain—so there didn't seem to be much reason to lay the burden of Mary's diagnosis on him and add to his concerns. Besides, Charles had a 50 percent chance of not having it. My father died in an automobile accident in his early 50s, so we'll never be able to find out if he was the transmitter. He probably was since my mother is in her 90s and going strong.

"I always thought it was better to live with denial and the assumption that everything would be fine. That's why I never mentioned this to my son, Robert. If you figure the odds, my chances are 50/50. Robert has a 25 percent chance, and his children only have a 12.5 percent chance, pretty small—so I've just kept it to myself.

"Yes, I've been worried about my brother Charles. I hoped it was Parkinsonism, but it did begin to look like what I remember of Mary. There's nothing you can do about Huntington's, so what would have been the point of telling him my suspicions? I'm not sure there's any point even now. If you could treat it, that would be a different matter.

"As for me, the last 25 years since Mary died have been good ones. I've watched Robert grow up and become successful. My wife and I have been happily married, my law practice has done better than I deserved, and I've had time to be active in civic organizations. Do you think I could have done better had I known that I wouldn't come down with Huntington's disease? Would it have been better if I knew I would get it when I was 40, or 50, or 60? I doubt it. It would have been a terrible burden to bear. In fact, I don't want to have that new genetic test, even now.

"While it would be unusually late for me to develop the symptoms, I realize that it's still possible. Of course, if I don't have the gene, my children and grandchildren don't have it either. But if they want to find out, they'll just have to have the test themselves. I want to live just as I have done.

"Of course, I could have encouraged Robert not to have children by his first wife. But there was no definitive test available only those few years ago. He might even have listened, but then he would not have had the pleasure of watching them grow up. And he would have had to carry that burden, too, for even longer than I. Now, he'll have to decide about this test for himself. If he has the gene, then he got it from me, and I will soon enough have the disease. I don't want to know about his test.

"I appreciate your concern, Dr. Gunderson. Thanks for listening to me. I guess I've kept it bottled up too long—you can tell—but it was better that way and I still think it is. Of course, you'll be keeping this information confidential, just between the two of us. As for Virginia, I don't care what that dame wants. If she's so desperate for a perfect baby, let her go adopt one or something. She's not my problem; the rest of the family is. Now that Charles has definite symptoms, I plan to talk with him. He can decide what to do about his family and a definitive test."

* * *

Mr. Smyth's Dilemma

What do you think about Mr. Smyth's position? Is living with denial a reasonable approach to a problem such as Huntington's? What are the consequences of such an approach for him and for his family?

Would he have been better if he had assumed the glass was half empty and acted as if he would come down with the disease? He could have increased his insurance, set his affairs in order, and taken a stable job with good benefits. Would this have been wise?

Should he have told his brother Charles? Did Charles have the right to know so he could make his own plans? Now that Charles is showing manifestations of the disease, is this the right time to tell him? Will it help Charles or his wife? What about Charles's children?

What would you have done if you had been in Mr. Smyth's shoes 20 to 25 years ago? What would you do if you were in his shoes now?

A direct genetic test for Huntington's is now available. An individual at risk for the disease can determine whether he or she carries the lethal gene. In some ways, this simplifies Mr. Smyth's problem. If Charles wants to know, he can find out for himself.

Of course, individuals will only get this test if they think they are at risk. Huntington's is a sufficiently rare condition that widespread screening would be unproductive. Does Mr. Smyth now have a duty that he did not have when there were no reliable tests for this disease?

Did Mr. Smyth have a duty to tell the others about Mary's condition and their own risks? What is the source of that duty? How would you resolve the conflicts between the rights of those who would want to know and of those who would not want to know. If you tell them about Mary, they will know they are at risk.

Try analyzing these issues with the utilitarian approach of the greatest happiness for the greatest number. What would have been the benefits of Mr. Smyth's telling the family about Mary's disease 25 years ago? Would Charles have been happier knowing of his 50 percent risk? How about his children, who will soon learn of their own risk? How about Robert? Would he have had children in his previous marriage had he known? Using this analysis, what should Mr. Smyth have done 25 years ago? What should he do now?

Now use a rights- and duties-based approach to answer the same questions. Do people have the right to all available genetic information about themselves? Do they have the right not to have such information? (According to a recent study, 25 percent of those at risk for Huntington's disease choose not to have a definitive test.) If people have the right to the information, who has the duty to give it? If an individual chooses not to know the information, do others (health care providers, relatives, friends, insurance companies) have the obligation not to disclose it?

If Robert tests positive, then his father also has the disease. How does the duty to divulge this information relate to the duty of confidentiality?

What do we think about the character of these people based on their decisions? Is Henry admirable for taking on the burden of knowledge? Or is he paternalistic and overbearing for doing so? Is Charles as weak as his brother portrays him? Should he have been more assertive in seeking information about Mary's death? What is a virtuous or admirable way to deal with a situation like this?

* * *

Charles's Response

"Thanks for telling me, Henry," Charles replies glumly when his brother breaks the news. "You know, I don't remember much about Mary. I was younger and it was kept very quiet. I always thought Mom was embarrassed about having her in a mental institution. But I remember some of the whispers and Mom's going to visit her. I think I've suspected this past year that I might have the same thing, but I was afraid to find out. I'll have the test to confirm it, but I feel I already know what I've got. At least now I know how to plan.

"And thanks for not burdening me with this information over all these years. It must have been a terrible responsibility for you to make that decision and to keep the secret, but it certainly made my life easier.

"I guess I'll have to tell my kids now. I hope they'll be able to cope. I guess their biggest decision will be whether or not to have the test themselves. They should have the same liberty I've had to live their lives without knowledge. It is hard to think that I would have been better off if I hadn't been born. I've had more than fifty wonderful years of life. I don't regret a day of it, not even this one. I hope this new test doesn't take away more choices than it gives.

"Anyway, you're a wonderful brother. Thanks."

Dr. Gunderson's Dilemma

"Dr. Gunderson, it's a counselor from the Genetics Counseling Center on the phone asking to speak with you about Charles Smyth. Would you like me to pull his chart?"

"No, thank you. . . . Gunderson speaking. Yes, Charles Smyth is my patient. Can you tell me what this is about?"

"I'm a genetics counselor at the Genetics Counseling Center. My patient is engaged to Robert Smyth. We were told that his Uncle Charles, who is under your care, has a neurological disorder, and we are checking to be sure it isn't any genetic disease that we should know about. I always like to be sure I'm accurate when I provide counseling.

"Hello . . . are you still there, Dr. Gunderson?"

* * *

Put yourself in Dr. Gunderson's position. What will you respond? You are bound to keep Charles Smyth's medical information confidential. What obligation do you have to his brother who shared the family history with you? Does his requesting confidentiality bind you to keep it? Does Virginia, who is not your patient nor even a member of the family, have any right to know? Will simply telling the counselor that the information is confidential in fact divulge the information? If you do not divulge the information, a baby may be born who, fifty years from now, could suffer and die from Huntington's.

* * *

Virginia's Response

"That bastard! Robert, do you realize what he's done to you and almost done to me! If you have that terrible disease you could become an invalid, a vegetable, or worse, a moving vegetable, in ten years. He allowed you to have children without even knowing, without being able to make an informed decision! They could have it, too! What right did he have to keep it all to himself? Who does he think he is, God? You had the right to make your own decisions.

"Poor Robert. You need to get tested right away. I don't know if I could stand watching you deteriorate. I am not the kind who could feed you and bathe you and treat you like an infant. Robert, what are we going to do?"

"Hold on, Virginia. If I test positive, what then? If the investors in the company we're about to launch get wind of it, do you think they'll invest? Our years of planning and development will go right down the drain. What then? Besides, I've got individual medical insurance. The insurance company may well cancel me if they find out. I've got to think this whole thing through. I'm not at all sure that I want to be tested."

* * *

Is Virginia's response unreasonable? How would you have responded if you suddenly found that your fiancé might have a progressive, crippling, dementing disease? Would you go through with marriage? Would you have children if they could be affected? Would your marriage depend on your fiancé's having the test? Is it morally acceptable to withhold information about your family history or test results from your fiancé? How do you draw the line between those things that must be disclosed and those that can be kept private?

In the next ten years, there will be an incredible expansion in the availability of genetic tests. These tests will be widely available, though given the expense of the tests, they will likely be inaccessible to many people. Is there a just way to apportion these scarce resources? Are there people who may not want them but nevertheless should have them? If the widespread availability of testing could benefit society, do individuals have a right to resist? How does confidentiality fit this picture?

Not only will there be tests for defects like Huntington's, but there will be new proposals to "improve the breed" by developing superior human beings. Can tests for genetic defects be sharply separated from tests for normal human capacities? Is genetic enhancement of human capacities legitimate? If we are on the verge of "designer human beings," should social controls be set in place? Is there a moral basis for refusing to control this powerful technology?

chapter
16
✻ ✻ ✻ ✻ ✻

The Perfect Rexford

via dot.dot.com total-mail <<<>>> routed cellular direct

September 18, 2020.

Mom, it's all decided, and we want you to be the first to know. The baby's name will be Shiboan Katherine. Don't you love it? It seems very regal to us and speaks to our Irish heritage. And we've agreed that she will be tall, with red hair and green eyes. Brad wants her to be cuddly as a youngster and independent as an adult. We thought about naming her Lucretia, but that went with a tall dark girl and it didn't sound like the rest of the family. It's amazing to sit in front of a computer and, starting with your own genetic characteristics, choose what you want for your child. The computer even shows her change as she grows up. It's very much like using those old online catalogs to buy my school clothes. I could see how they would look on me. We still need to negotiate the deafness issue. I hope the people at the Genomic Center will listen to us (pardon the metaphor!). Brad also is excited, and we're going to the Center next week to finalize the arrangements. We'll put the pictures on our website as soon as we have everything decided.

Love to dad,   Martha.

✻   ✻   ✻

"Brad," signed Martha, "I made the appointment for next Thursday at the Genomic Center. Can you make it? You have to be there to help to make the final decisions about the proper combinations of genes. Brad, this is so exciting. I can't imagine how mom and dad just left everything to chance and then prayed for the best. Honey, it is okay to do this, don't you think? We can afford to, and, if we're only going to have one child, she ought to be perfect.

Oh, Brad, I've dreamed about this baby for so long; I can't wait until next week."

* * *

Consider the following mostly fictional though plausible, "history":

Starting in the late 1980s, scientists began mapping all the genes in the human genome. The genes could be cloned and, by the 1990s, they could modify the genetic material of animals and clone them. By the turn of the millennium, scientists learned how to sort sperm into X-carrying and Y-carrying so it became easy, with simple insemination technology, to carry out parents' preference for a female or a male infant. As the technology for gene transfer and for the insertion of promoter and suppressor genes in animals was perfected, the demand to cure genetic defects became overwhelming. In 2007 restrictions on modifying human gene structure were lifted and the technology was first used to cure cystic fibrosis by gene insertion. Treatment for Tay-Sachs disease and Huntington's chorea followed shortly. It was soon regarded as unethical to withhold a simple procedure like gene transfer when it was possible to cure such devastating conditions. About the same time it became possible to alter the genes which predisposed to colon or breast cancer, thus enhancing the lives of those predisposed to these diseases.

By 2015 the techniques of gene elimination, substitution, promotion, and suppression were commonly used to promote health and to prevent disease. They were expensive, but the National Health and Disease Prevention Agency (NHDPA) after much debate reached a consensus that, not only were these techniques important for decreasing disease and suffering, but they were also greatly to society's economic benefit. The cost of cure was far less than the cost of treatment.

With these dramatic advances in the applications of the new molecular biology came the ability to produce "designer babies." The combinations of genes for eye and hair color, and for height had been identified. By 2020 some of the many genes contributing to intelligence or musical or athletic ability were discovered and could potentially be modified. The processes for the modification of the multiple alleles were not completely perfected. They were going to be expensive, but they were on the verge of becoming available. The NHDPA refused, of course, to cover such elective enhancement procedures, but there were fewer and fewer obstacles for those who could afford it.

* * *

In the year 2020, Brad Rexford was 38, had recently sold his first successful software firm and was starting another. He had married Martha 14 years before when they had each been in graduate school in Boston. Martha was now the vice president of a prestigious New York bank supervising its Diverse

Abilities Compliance Assurance program. The fact that Martha had a hereditary form of deafness helped her to relate to the needs of variously abled workers.

Alert to the rapid developments in biotechnology, the Rexfords had put off having their child until the required technology became available. One day Brad found the Genomic Center's Website whose home page opened with the following banner:

The Genomic Center

Better Babies Through Molecular Biology

Why run the risk of breast cancer when the genes which predispose to this condition can be eliminated? Do you have a family history of colon cancer? Are you a carrier? You need not pass this fear to your children. Why have your children worry when we can now eliminate the disease—and the fear?

Modern molecular biology now enables us to avoid many of the ills that flesh is heir to and enables you to give your children their very best chance of a healthy, satisfying life.

Consult With Us When You Are Planning
Your Next Child
Perhaps we can help

Since The Genomic Center starts each embryo with the parents' own genetic material, your children are assured of having all the genetic advantages of their parents, and a wonderful opportunity to move beyond them.

---

* * *

After spending hours at the computer filling out an extensive, detailed history about all the diseases and conditions of brothers, sisters, aunts, cousins, and, of course, parents and grandparents, Martha made a personal appointment for herself and Brad. The Genomic Center was located on the 32nd floor of the GenXX Building on Madison Avenue. The offices spoke of the future with the most stylish decor. The staff had obviously read the questionnaire carefully since they had a sign language interpreter on hand for the first interview.

As Martha retold the story, Dr. Knowles introduced himself and, rather pretentiously, began by telling her that her type of congenital deafness was located on gene 7, seventeen telemeres from the centromere. While he would have to recheck her chromosomes and Brad's, the form of deafness that she had was usually dominant. Since there were no other deaf members in her family, it probably represented a new mutation. Brad's deafness had a different genetic cause, which explained the variations in hearing ability in his family. Dr. Knowles said, that by using fluorescent dye techniques and the newly developed ultramicro laser only recently available at the center, it was possible to delete segment 7.504b and insert a small promoter gene. That should prevent deafness in the child. Although the number of individuals on whom this had been done was still very small, he believed there was roughly a 70 percent chance of eliminating deafness in the baby. He ended by admitting that the laser technique was not yet perfect, but then not everything in life was—at least not yet.

Only when he finally paused could they tell him that they hadn't come to the center to have a hearing baby. She and Brad said they preferred to have a child just like themselves, only better. They were very satisfied with their lives and were both leaders in the deaf community. Designing a hearing child would be an affront to everything they stood for. Martha had been president of the American Sign Language Institute, and was still active on the board. Brad was chair of the Development Committee for the Association for the Hard of Hearing which was in the midst of a $25 million campaign for renovation of its New York headquarters. Although it wasn't directly relevant to their visit, they also explained their reasons for rejecting cochlear implants for themselves and for any children they might have.

They explained that, although they hoped and expected their little girl to be deaf, they wanted to give her every advantage in life. They repeated their desire that she be tall and slender with red hair and green eyes. They also said that, though they were unclear about progress in modifying genes for personality and intelligence, they were confident about her genetic endowment, although they would consider any enhancements the center might offer. In terms of personality, they repeated their preference that she lean toward the self-confident and assertive side. They explained that these were the reasons for their consultation and asked what the center could do to help.

Dr. Knowles became very uncomfortable at this point in the conversation. He admitted that they had not designed the Web form to accommodate this preference. The center had always assumed people would be working to eliminate hereditary deafness. He bluntly admitted that he was surprised. It was very difficult for him, he said, because it is not why he went into genetics. He had studied the molecular biology of reproduction in order to prevent disease, to help families with bad genes have normal children.

Yet he saw their arguments. He recognized that the technology was available. The process starts just like in vitro fertilization with harvesting the woman's eggs. Then the man's Y-sperm is separated from the X-sperm. The Xs are used to fertilize the eggs, which generate female embryos. The tricky part is the laser surgery to implant the red hair gene and the genes for green eyes. There will be a surplus of embryos, but only one will be implanted. It may not take, but there'll be others ready.

The genetic analysis of the embryos will show which of them has the gene for Martha's type of deafness.

From this point in the conversation, Martha can recount Dr. Knowles's words from memory:

"Here is the tough decision. You've said you prefer a deaf child. Do you want us to destroy the embryos with the potential for hearing? Are you sure you don't want us to implant a hearing one? Or do you not want to know? Since your type of deafness is autosomal dominant, each embryo has a 50/50 chance it will not be deaf. We could pick an embryo at random and implant it.

"Frankly, I am deeply troubled at the idea of my contributing to a project of deliberately bringing a deaf child into the world. My work is devoted to preventing such infirmities. It would ease my conscience considerably if you would agree to implanting an embryo at random with respect to hearing. Then I wouldn't be creating a deaf child.

"I have no problem with enhancing a child's quality of life, whether or not she is deaf. You seem to think that red hair and green eyes are an enhancement. It's a matter of taste, perhaps, but it poses no moral problem for me. You want a girl; why not? But choosing an embryo for implantation *because* it is deaf, that may be outside the boundaries of my tolerance. I have to give that a lot of thought."

*   *   *

Granted that what the Rexfords have requested is not available now, but it probably will be soon. The history of technological development shows that once techniques are available, they will be used, and not necessarily for the purposes for which they were originally intended. Mapping the human genome was undertaken to understand the genetic components and causes of disease and to identify the genes which predisposed a person to particular conditions. But the same research will open possibilities beyond the imagination, much less control, of those who launched this study.

The control of technology poses significant ethical challenges. In one way, technology is morally neutral; the same devices can be used for good or ill. On the other hand, however, some technologies seem to invite destructive uses. Nuclear energy, for example, is suspect because it was first used in weapons. One way of dealing with the morally legitimate uses of genetic technology is to divide the issues between the public and the private. If we have difficulty agreeing what it is right to do, we might be able to agree who is to decide. Some decisions should be made by society, while others are left to individuals.

As discussed in Chapter 18, drawing the distinction between public and private morality is one of the most challenging aspects of contemporary medical ethics. For example, the controversy over abortion is largely an argument over whether abortion is a public or private matter. In these discussions, private issues are those in which society is willing to tolerate a wide variety of individual choices. In matters of sexual practice, for example, our society has generally decided to tolerate wide variation. While people may find the sexual practices of others morally repulsive, few of us are prepared to regulate such sexual expression. Spousal beating, on the other hand, used to be regarded as a private matter, but most of us now regard it as deserving public restriction. Practices which we once tolerated, if not approved, are no longer socially tolerated, and vice versa.

Drawing the line between the public and the private involves the vexed question of the relation between law and morality. Some of our laws plainly enforce moral standards; laws against murder, theft, and fraud are obvious examples. Yet the morality of the law itself restricts the scope of its operation. In the United States, we place such a high moral value on free speech that it is very difficult to prosecute those guilty of deliberate slander. The morality of our law restricts the law's application to what we have decided are public matters.

Consider whether the uses of genetic technology that the Rexfords plan are public or private matters:

The Public Issues

The Human Genome Project has been funded by the National Science Foundation, and many other aspects of basic genetic research and therapeutic techniques are funded by this and other agencies of the U.S. government. The funding was justified by the potential this knowledge has for preventing genetic diseases. But the very same technology can be used to satisfy the Rexfords, and specific techniques and genetic agents spun off from the research can be patented. For example, a group of scientists has patented a genetically modified strain of mice. Since this knowledge was generated largely at public expense, should the government control who benefits from the knowledge? Should it insure that all citizens have equal access to its benefits? Should all citizens enjoy all the benefits, right down to the Rexfords' (frivolous?) choice of a red-haired child? Is there an effective way to limit or control what benefits are provided? Should researchers be allowed to profit individually from publicly sponsored research? Will giving government a role in controlling this technology give it an unjustly large role in controlling our lives?

The Private Issues

The Rexfords want a baby with certain characteristics, they can afford it, and their preferences do not interfere in an obvious way with anyone else's well-being. It is possible that these are morally neutral choices. It is also possible to disapprove of these choices, yet regard them as private; that is, choices we are prepared to socially tolerate if not personally approve. We might argue that genetic technology, like any other, can be misused, but we will leave it to individuals to use or misuse it as they see fit. Without clear evidence that what the Rexfords are proposing is morally wrong, is there anything to discuss? Consider some of the possible issues of moral concern:

- Is it a distortion of the human condition to want a child made to order? Is it vanity for parents to want a child like themselves, even to the extent of wanting a deaf child? Are we in danger of turning our children into consumer commodities? These are moral issues for the virtue ethics tradition. If these practices violate the rights of future generations, they are issues for the deontological tradition of duties and rights. If they will lead to reduced human welfare in the future, they are issues for utilitarians.
- Can researchers maintain moral neutrality and leave the decisions to the parents? How can scientists retain a personal morality and still allow their work to be used in whatever way others see fit? Compare this with the moral situation of those who worked on nuclear research in the 1950s. How should scientists draw the line on parental requests that they could not accept?

Put yourself in the position of the decision-makers in this case.

As a parent, what boundaries would you place on your own choices? Is it acceptable to choose your child's hair or eye color? Gender? Personality type, intelligence, or talents? Other characteristics, such as deafness, that are generally regarded as handicaps? If you make these choices, are you thinking of your children as commodities, as good things to have in your life, or are you thinking of the well-being of the children themselves? Are these choices very different from the choice of a good school? When you answer these questions, do your answers rest on an ethical theory or are they your current moral intuitions or feelings?

As a researcher, what boundaries would you place on the uses of the science and technology you had discovered? How would you argue against the charge that you are imposing your own views and unethically preventing others from exercising their own moral judgment? Is it even possible to control the uses that others make of your discoveries? When you answer these questions, do your answers rest on an ethical theory or are they your current moral intuitions or feelings?

Finally, as a legislator, what boundaries would you place on the use of science and technology? How would you argue against the charge that you are imposing your own views and unethically preventing others from exercising moral judgment? Is it practically possible to regulate the spread of technology, given that people can go anywhere in the world to get treatments they want? Again, when you answer these questions about the moral scope and power of the law, do your answers rest on an ethical theory or are they your current moral intuitions or feelings?

PART
V

HEALTH CARE REFORM AND
ETHICAL THEORY

chapter
17
✳ ✳ ✳ ✳ ✳

Affordable Health Care

"He wants us to have a draft of the health plan by the end of the week so that he can present it at the AMA convention." Joe McLaughlin is a 36-year-old lawyer on loan to the presidential campaign from a big Washington consulting firm. "He says he'll shoot us if we come up with a disaster like Hillary's plan, but he liked some of her basic principles. My notes say that he wants to be sure the speech touches on his basic themes: universality, affordability, quality, and responsibility.

"Hillary and her Clinton Health Plan of 1995 tried to do too much, too fast, and for too many people. As soon as her plan came out, every group in D.C. started lobbying for its own agenda. No one was willing to work for the compromises needed to achieve its goals. The present administration fell into exactly the same trap; they failed by trying to keep everyone happy. O'Brien, one of his speech writers, sent over a draft titled 'The Affordable Health Care Act of 2005.' The boss wants it at the top of his legislative agenda right after the elections. He wants us to put together a health policy panel to mark up O'Brien's draft."

George LaFarge, an enthusiastic young attorney on loan to the campaign from Hogan-Pickering, agrees: "I'll have Liz get a panel together for Thursday. She'll send out a draft so they look it over before they come. Let's read it aloud now to get some feel for how it sounds."

Joe reads the draft in his most presidential voice:

The Affordable Health Care Act of 2005

Doctors—ladies and gentlemen. It is a great honor to give the opening address at this meeting. The American Medical Association has always been known for its leadership, pushing the frontiers to deliver optimum health care for all our citizens. Yet it is plain to all of you that our great health care system has many problems. Today I would like to present you with an outline, a first proposal, for achieving the fair, just, and comprehensive health system that we all desire. This plan incorporates the statement of freedoms for which Franklin D. Roosevelt was so justly famous, especially freedom from fear and freedom from want, to which our country has added freedom of choice, and to which our administration will add freedom to act responsibly.

Here are some of the issues a health plan for all Americans must address:

- The public feels *insecure* about paying for health care. People feel locked into jobs because they fear losing health insurance if they change employers.

- Our present system is so *complex* that people don't understand what coverage they have, what is included and what is excluded. We waste everyone's time and money with bureaucratic attempts to micromanage the system. Our new system must be simple, understandable, and comprehensive.

- *Costs* must be contained. America has the most expensive health care system in the world, and yet our people are not as healthy as people in other industrialized countries that spend much less money. There must be ways to control the ever-expanding health care costs while maintaining our excellent quality and extending our wonderful care to the whole population.

- No plan that constrains *freedom* within the medical system will ever be acceptable. As the recent crisis in managed care shows, Americans have always valued their freedom, especially the freedom to choose their medical care.

- But with choice comes *responsibility*. We must depend on our citizens to make responsible choices and our great medical profession to assure that individuals choose among reasonable alternatives.

Since this is a democracy in which every person is equal and has certain inalienable rights, it is our belief that everyone should have the right to basic health coverage. However, with rights come obligations, and therefore we believe that every citizen also has the obligation to carry and pay for that insurance. If people can't drive a car without insurance, they shouldn't be able to walk around without medical coverage. No one should be able to take a free ride on the system.

Our proposal will require both the employer and the individual to contribute to their health insurance premium. If everyone has to contribute to health care, companies will build it into the cost of business. It is a further feature of my proposal that the self-employed and those few people who are too wealthy to need to work will have a health insurance premium as part of their income tax. We'll provide for the desperately poor through a tax rebate for health care. Universal coverage prevents shifting costs from the uninsured to others who are bearing the burden of the system. Under my leadership there will be universal health coverage and universal payment for that coverage.

The issue of health care demands a new level of realism and maturity on the part of the general public. While society provides roads and public transportation, we accept the fact that not everyone gets to ride in the same comfort. Some drive ordinary cars, others drive luxury vehicles, while still others take public transit. When we talk about health care, everyone needs basic care, but the amenities, the things that are clearly elective, those we can leave to the marketplace.

For any system such as mine to work, it must draw a firm line between medically required and optional care. Here is a list of procedures for which I oppose insurance payment:

- Cosmetic surgery, tummy tucks, face lifts, breast augmentation, and other procedures that are not required for health.
- Fertility treatments and in vitro fertilization. We in the United States should not contribute to the world's population crisis.
- Everyday medications: Maalox for sour stomachs, aspirin for headaches, herbs, vitamins, so-called natural remedies, and all the symptomatic treatments that do not cure disease but merely make people feel better.
- All other unproven alternative therapies such as acupuncture, chiropractic, and special diets. We will withhold payment until they meet the accepted medical tests of efficacy and safety.

I know that these limits are challenging and the special interests will oppose them. While it may seem strange that I address these remarks to you, I need the support of the medical leadership in the AMA to limit health care at both ends of life. It is not a fair distribution of health care resources that some in our country get everything they want while others lack some basic things they need. I need your help to gather the political will to work for the good of society as a whole.

We must work to be fair to every generation: the old, the middle, and the young. In particular, we should limit the care of those at the extreme ends of the scale—those very old and those very young—who consume a vastly disproportionate share of health care efforts. There is much work to be done on the details, but suppose at age 75 each individual received a credit of $200,000 on a medical ATM card for their future lifetime of medical care. This allowance would permit everyone the freedom of choice about how they spend their last days. For example, individuals who have a stroke or a heart attack could receive the acute care they needed. As they recovered, they could get appropriate rehabilitation. The patient, with their family, could choose how to spend the resources. They could spend the money quickly in an intensive care unit, less rapidly on a hospital ward, slowly in a nursing care facility, or even more slowly at home with assistance. Most, of course, would choose some combination of these. The patient gets to make a responsible choice. When the money is all spent, the patient receives only comfort care, but no major medical testing and no major interventions. If someone dies with money left over, the family gets to keep half, and the other half returns to the U.S. Treasury.

I propose a similar limitation on care at the beginning of life. High-technology resuscitation and treatment of small babies should only be permitted when clinical research has documented that the rate of high-quality survival is better than 50 percent. For example, nothing other than comfort care should be done for infants less than one and a half pounds. Currently each nursery makes up its own rules. Often different physicians within a given nursery have their own biases. We believe that this is unfair to the babies, their families, and society. Even if a few of these very small babies were to survive to lead happy lives, the large number that absorb resources and then die, and the even larger number who survive with mental retardation, cerebral palsy, blindness, or other handicaps is a huge burden on the families and on society as a whole. When their baby is struggling for survival, parents are under too much stress to make responsible decisions. Setting firm national guidelines is to everyone's advantage.

I also propose rationing of costly innovations. If we eliminate heart transplants for those over age 70, for example, we could save a lot of money. I propose to prohibit bone marrow transplants for patients over 50 and kidney transplants for those over age 65. We know that some will be excluded who would have done well with the transplant, but we have to have fairness and some equality in this new system, and we can't provide everything to everyone and still keep it affordable.

We agree with those who claim that technological improvements, while they are the best part of our healthcare system, nevertheless drive up costs. And we say the era of unlimited spending is over. While continuing to foster the research which has made the United States the leader of the world by increasing the funding of both basic and clinical research, our administration will deny payment for experimental treatments until the research studies show that the increase in costs is justified by the improvement in society's health and well-being. Faster MRI scans can produce beautiful images, but it is not clear that the increase in cost is justified by the benefits for health.

We are committed, however, to using some of the money saved for careful studies of molecular biology: technology for transplanting genes and the applications of stem cell research is extremely promising. At first new therapies will only be obtainable as part of carefully controlled studies. Until they are documented to provide a dramatic improvement in the quality of life for a majority of the individuals receiving the therapy, they won't be covered by insurance or available to individuals outside the studies.

Dramatic, even radical, medical care reform is our only hope. We have to begin to make policies based on what is best for society as a whole, not what is best for a few individuals.

Ladies and gentlemen of the AMA, at this historic juncture we need your help. Society needs your wisdom and cooperation. Now is the time to provide every citizen of this great nation with the best health care that members of your association know how to deliver. If I am elected, I pledge to work together with you to make this country a model for the world and an even better place to live and to raise our children. God bless you all for all you already do and for your help as we work together toward an even healthier society.

"Well, O'Brien's got us off to a start. But presenting his plan to the AMA is like waving a red cape in front of an angry bull," concludes George LaFarge. "We'll have the deep thinkers run through it at the meeting Thursday and see what they have to say."

* * *

What do you have to say about the ideas embodied in this speech? Any complex public policy proposal has many political and economic aspects, but try to evaluate the proposal primarily from a moral point of view.

Does society have a duty to provide health care for its members? How is that duty derived? Is it included in the social contract, an obligation of society to protect its members against threats to their lives? Is it derived from the fundamental value of health care in our culture? If so, why have people in the United States taken so long to notice that health care is a fundamental value that requires public provision?

Does the plan adequately address the utilitarian goal of providing the greatest happiness for the greatest number, or does it leave too much room for entrenched special interests? Does utilitarianism require the rationing this plan includes? Does rationing force us to overlook too many individual preferences and differences?

Is the plan fair in allocating the burdens and benefits of modern medicine? Is it fair to deny or limit care to the elderly, who have contributed to the medical system all their lives? Is it fair to deny or limit medical care to fragile newborns, the most vulnerable members of society? Are the burdens of paying for the system fairly shared among individuals, employers, and the government?

Is the universal provision of health care a mark of a caring and virtuous society? Should one argue that the moral quality of a society is revealed by the care it provides for its most burdened members?

The following discussion of the health care panel is designed to give you a taste of the moral and political complexity of health care reform.

*   *   *

"This is quite a gang you've gathered for the session, George," begins Joe McLaughlin. "We'd better start with introductions. These people have all heard of one another, but some of them may never have met."

"Good idea, Joe. Let's go around the table: Jerry Wallerstein on my left is a consultant on health care and other benefits to the steelworkers and several other unions. Next to him is Marge Forrest, director of the Health Policy Institute's think tank. Devon Malachi is on the staff at the Bioethics Institute. Heather Sterling joins us from the American Business Institute, and Bill Glass is a political consultant sent over by the party. Che Quin is sitting in on this session. He's a graduate student in public policy doing an internship with me."

"I think it's a very strong opening," rasps Wallerstein in his gravelly voice. "Perhaps it's too strong for the doctors; they may need some of these pills sugar-coated. But our members respond to the New Deal and FDR. That language works for our people. With all the downsizing that's been going on, our members are afraid of losing their jobs, but even more frightened of losing health coverage. There are jobs these days, but a lot of them don't offer coverage at all, and even the ones that do have a waiting period before the coverage kicks in. It's hard to get coverage for preexisting conditions.

"Our members will support universal coverage; we've been fighting for it for decades. What makes your boss think he'll get it this time around? How are you going to get the doctors, insurers, and the small business people on board? They've always resisted it. I'm not sure the universal payment part of the plan will convince them.

"From unions' point of view, of course, we think the fast food restaurants and some small businesses are always complaining that they cannot afford to contribute to health insurance, but they also claimed they could not afford it when Congress raised the minimum wage. They'll all raise the price of fries by a nickel. It's not the big deal they make it out to be."

"Before we settle in to another rehash of the politics of getting something passed," Marge Forrest interrupts, "let's remind ourselves of the moral premise that society is obligated to provide fundamental benefits for all its members. That makes health care a basic right.

"Alone among industrialized, democratic countries, the U.S. has failed to fulfill this obligation to its people. This country has opted for an insurance model in which each individual or group takes responsibility for covering any medical catastrophes of their members. We modified that in 1965 with Medicaid for the very poor and Medicare for the elderly. Yet millions of children lack any health coverage. We ought to be ashamed. Medical care is a basic social good that should be fairly and equitably distributed. It is like public highways or public schools. The government has poured uncountable billions into the public highway system, and the only objections are from people who want more. The health of the public is an even more basic need. People should have access to a physician and to a hospital when they need it. There should be no worry about the cost. People should receive the medicines they need.

"Not only is such an approach superior to what we have, it actually works. Britain, for example, spends less than half percapita of what we do. Their infant mortality is lower than ours and their longevity is higher. It doesn't matter that patients can't get a scan on demand or can't get a bad hip replaced for a year. The numbers on the bottom line argue that their health care is, on balance, better than ours. Their system seems to have two advantages. Because it treats every resident equally, it is fairer and more democratic. Because it is cheaper and gets better results, it is also more efficient. That sounds to me like a win-win situation; better morality and better medicine."

"Could I put in a good word for some political realism?" George LaFarge begins. "The speech we're working over is about as far out as anyone can go in the U.S. The everyday rationing that goes on in Britain would never be tolerated in this country. It's not even tolerated there. Those who can afford it go to their private doctors and private hospitals. If their egalitarian system is making them so happy, why do so many Brits get their care outside the system? All the moral satisfaction of knowing that everyone is equal and shares the same system will not offset the delays and frustrations that come with a huge national bureaucracy. While it's plain that these systems improve health on average, averages are not people. Many wealthy Britons feel better that they can go outside the system; the same would happen here.

"Before you start screaming 'sell out,' I'd like to remind you of the morality of political realism. It sounds terribly moral when Wallerstein invokes utilitarian principles of equality and happiness for the greatest number, and Marge's plea for a right to health care is noble indeed. But I don't see that practicality is at war with genuine morality. Some say that politics is the art of the possible. I think genuine morality deals with the possible as well. In fact, I think that pie-in-the-sky moral theorizing is actually immoral. The point of real morality is not to think about things but to change them for the better. Moral idealism that does not work is not a higher morality."

"I know you folks invited me to be the spoiler at this party," began Heather

Sterling from the American Business Institute. "But I liked those parts of the speech that spoke to personal responsibility. It's an element of morality that's been missing in the conversation so far. Utilitarians, so concerned about happiness and welfare, are soft on responsibility. The Kantians, betraying their founder, talk about the right to health care with little reference to responsibility. I think personal responsibility for health and health care is morally significant and needs to be a part of any acceptable plan.

"The Institute has a proposal that provides universal coverage and still preserves personal responsibility. We agree that everyone should carry insurance, but insurance should only cover catastrophic medical bills. Coverage would be provided either by government or private companies. Each individual over age 18 would be personally responsible for the first $2,000 of medical expenses each year.

"There would be a separate program for children. After the first $2,000, insurance would pay 90 percent. When an individual has paid $5,000 or a family $10,000, insurance will pay 100 percent. There would have to be a safety net for the poor, of course, and for those with large families.

"Under this proposal, when someone goes to a physician with a headache and the physician suggests a brain scan, instead of saying 'When?' patients would be forced to ask how much it's going to cost, since they would have to pay for each of these tests until they had laid out the $2,000. Patients would think twice about how bad that headache really is.

"When people get colds, they can go to the doctor, be examined, and get a prescription, but they have to pay for the whole thing. A cold or the flu will usually last a week under a physician's care, but seven days if they take care of it themselves. Every time someone's arthritis flares up, they're going to have to take aspirin or whatever unless they want to pay the physician's fee and the costs of the newest and perhaps unproven treatment. This proposal aims at establishing a genuine catastrophic insurance system; it only pays when expenses go beyond what most people can afford.

"Our consultants say that a lot of money is saved when patients are aware of and have a stake in the costs of tests and treatments. They believe it will save money. Better than that, it fosters responsibility. The universal provision of care may make people happy, but it also makes them lazy. Insurance theory has a fancy term for it: *moral hazard*. When people take out an insurance policy on something, they begin to take less personal responsibility for the item because 'it's covered.' If we are going to treat individuals like adults and give them freedom to choose, we have to hold them accountable for the choices they make. A pure insurance system like this encourages autonomy and moral responsibility. This system would be morally superior to the social equality of a nationalized system. It would also be at least as efficient because so many small claims would be paid out of pocket. If this system saves the money we think it will, it passes George's test for practical morality. We'd like to emphasize the personal responsibility parts of the speech."

"Hold on, Heather," interrupts Devon Malachi. "There is a danger of getting bogged down in the details. Both you conservatives and the liberals who worked on Hillary's plan have too great a love for complicated systems. I'm glad there's not too much of that in the speech.

"Can we move onto the hard part—the issue of rationing?" he continues. "We've just heard a proposal to constrain the day-to-day demands on the system, but we also have to find a way to place some constraints on the end-of-life costs. Although patients and families say, 'I don't want to die like that, hooked up to machines or stuck in a hospital,' when decisions have to be made, they want everything done. Physicians are reluctant to say no, because they accept the patient's right to decide, because of the threats from the malpractice system, and at least partially from the financial incentives to provide more.

"I liked the part of the speech that comes to grips with this issue. We've got to put caps on spending for both the very young and the very old. The greatest happiness for the greatest number comes from spending money where it can make the most difference. That is both fair and efficient. I don't know how politically realistic this is, George, but I'm sure it's both morally significant and fiscally necessary."

"May I raise a question?" Che Quin asked tentatively. "In my culture, we venerate the elderly, whether healthy or sick. My parents are very proud of their accomplishments since coming to this country, and they're fiercely independent. They would want the best and the longest life for my aged grandparents if something should happen to them. They have saved for such an eventuality. While others have bought larger houses, bigger cars, and gone on vacations, my family has lived simply. If something were to happen to a family member and he outlived his medical allotment, would the candidate's plan prevent our taking advantage of the most sophisticated treatment? Could my family continue to support him with whatever he needed out of their own money?"

"That is an important question, Che," Malachi mutters. "Our talk of individual responsibility implies that people will have freedom to spend their money beyond the limits imposed by the system. Yet, once we allow that camel's nose in the tent, we've blown the equality that is an important part of the proposal. Also, doctors and other providers will quickly migrate to the private-pay parts of medical care, and the public sector will quickly become overcrowded and understaffed. Yet, in a free society, I don't see any way around the dilemma."

Bill Glass is the last to comment. "I think these proposals and counterproposals will bring nothing but trouble in the election. You can see from our own discussion that thinking about this stuff quickly gets incredibly complicated. The voters can't deal with the complications you policy wonks love. You people forget some basic truths, and, when the public remembers them, they turn against all these fancy proposals. Keep these facts in mind: Longevity in the United States, for those who reach age 65, is the highest in the world. Reforms in the Social Security system in the 1960s virtually eliminated poverty in the elderly. Longevity is highly correlated with income. Americans, especially the relatively well-off older people who actually vote in this country, are not particularly unhappy about their health care. They've got Social Security and Medicare. There's not a politician alive who is going to touch those programs. And old folks get suspicious that all these big ideas are going to undermine their security. My advice is: forget about it. Leave it alone. It ain't broke too bad; trying to fix it may make it worse.

"Above all, it won't help us win the election. That's my morality."

* * *

Wallerstein reports that people in the labor movement respond to the rhetoric of the New Deal. But given the religious and moral diversity of contemporary America, should health care reform rest on broad political principles such as freedom from fear or freedom to choose, or should it be based on a more concrete pragmatism? Is it morally better to settle for a system that works or are we obliged to strive for a morally ideal system?

Is Marge Forrest correct that health care is a basic right? What is the moral basis for this right (see the discussion of rights in Chapter 18)? How does a right to health care relate to the political liberties that our society also values? If government insures health care, should people lose the "right" to smoke cigarettes?

Is George LaFarge correct in arguing that there is a morality to political pragmatism? Is there a moral danger in trying to ground practical issues directly in moral theory?

How do you evaluate Heather Sterling's argument that comprehensive health coverage will make people lazy and diminish personal responsibility? Is there a moral hazard in comprehensive medical care?

Is Devon Malachi right in arguing that rationing is morally required? Which kinds of rationing systems are morally acceptable and which kinds are not acceptable? Is it fair to base rationing on age as the speech proposes? Is it acceptable to ration care on the basis of degree of physical handicap? Mental handicap?

Is Malachi's response to Che Quin correct in accepting an inevitable conflict between the equality imposed by a universal health care system and the freedom to make individual and family choices?

Is Bill Glass right in saying that all the talk about reforming American health care is useless moralizing because there is no deep political will in the electorate to change the present arrangements?

Finally, if you could make just one change in America's health care arrangements, what would that be? How would it relate to the moral and structural issues raised in this chapter?

chapter 18

Ethical Theory and Medical Ethics

Defining Morals and Ethics

In both popular and professional language, the terms *moral* and *ethical* are used in several senses. Public officials are sometimes guilty of "unethical" behavior, while people who violate a law dealing with sexual activity are arrested on "morals" charges. College courses on ethics are often taught by moral philosophers. Although *moral* is sometimes used as a word of praise, as in "She is a very moral person," on other occasions it has a wider and more neutral meaning, as in "Euthanasia is a moral issue."

In this and the following chapter we use *moral* to refer to the actions or activities for which a certain kind of praise or blame is awarded. Morally good or right actions are marked, for example, by courage, wisdom, balance, or fairness, while morally bad or wrong actions are characterized by opposite qualities. We use *morality* to refer to the collection of an individual's or a society's moral actions.

We praise people for many things, such as their intelligence or athletic ability. Some people excel in sports or in school primarily on native ability. While we admire or even envy such people, we have a different kind of admiration for people who bring certain personal attributes to whatever they do. As the cliché says, "It matters not whether you win or lose, it's how you play the game," and we might add, *how* you make decisions.

The outer box of Figure 18–1 diagrams all human activity. Moral activity falls inside the circle; activity or behavior outside the moral circle is non-moral or morally neutral, neither good nor bad. We do innumerable non-moral things all the time, such as breathe, chew gum, and sleep.

The borders of morally significant activity are, however, notoriously hard to define. They are themselves matters of substantial controversy. Are cigarette smoking, taxpaying, or gambling morally neutral and indifferent? There is controversy about where these examples would fit into our picture; some peo-

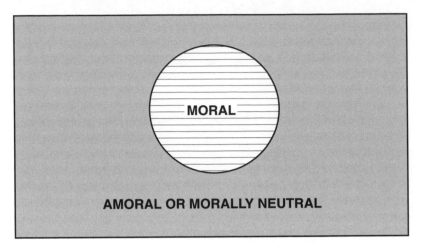

Figure 18-1

ple claim that smoking, for example, is just a neutral habit, while others say that, because it is harmful to health, the decision to smoke is part of one's moral makeup.

Moral activity is not exotic; we act as moral people every day. Discussion or argument about morality is also very ordinary. We evaluate the actions of others, and we think critically about ourselves. We are concerned about how people evaluate us and even more about how we really are. As we use the word, ethics is the discussion about and theory of morality. Whenever we discuss morals, we appeal either implicitly or explicitly to theories or principles justifying our judgments. Ethics, as Figure 18-2 shows, is like a grid that fits over our moral activity.

Defining ethics and morality as we do makes some matters a little clearer. For example, failing a course in ethics need not be a moral disgrace. In fact, people may fail for admirable reasons, such as missing classes and assignments to care for a sick parent. Furthermore, taking a course in ethics may help people see the issues of morality a little more clearly than they otherwise might have. There is no guarantee, naturally, that a course will produce better people, nor is a medical school requirement in medical ethics likely to improve dramatically the morality of those who take the course. Defining the terms this way also accounts for the fact that some philosophers who know a lot about ethical theory are not admirable people and that some morally upstanding people know very little ethical theory.

The case studies in this book, so far as possible, treat you as a participant in

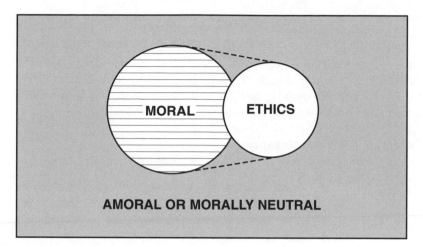

Figure 18-2

moral decision making. They also help you to realize that discussing these matters makes you an ethical theorist whether or not you relish that role. The theories we are about to discuss are not merely abstract possibilities or bright ideas from far away and long ago. They are ways in which people actually discuss with each other what should be done and also ways to think about ourselves and how we act.

Throughout the cases we have involved you in the process of making moral decisions. We hope and expect that thinking about the reasons for making decisions, and understanding how others might think about them, will help in making better decisions. Ethics, as we are concerned with it, is not a theory for outsiders to moral decision-making. Since morality is not a spectator sport, ethics, as we deal with it, is a theory of morality for participants.

The participant perspective is incompatible, we think, with relativism. In its simplest form, moral relativism holds that the rightness of an action is relative to each individual—right action is what each person thinks is right. A social version of the theory holds that right action is what each society regards as right. Philosophers have advanced some excellent arguments against relativism, but arguments are often ineffective in a classroom that enjoys a safe distance from real decisions and in which relativism often passes for tolerance. We hope that the virtual reality of the cases in this book will reduce the safe distance people sometimes put between themselves and real decisions. The cases provoke readers to think what they would do and what justifications they would offer. We hope this approach, while not itself an argument, will serve to dispel relativism.

Ethics, therefore, is not as separate from morality as our previous statements might have suggested. What people do is strongly influenced by what they think, and how they think is much influenced by what they do. All of us are involved in both morality and ethics. We have all been speaking ethics for a long time; reviewing ethical theory should help us to speak better.

Public and Private Morality

Just as distinguishing between ethics and morality can clarify our discussion, distinguishing public from private morality can save a great deal of confusion (see Figure 18–3).

The problems of medical ethics are especially vexing because they exist on the border between public and private morality. Unlike issues of racism or capital punishment, which are clearly public, and attitudes of personal respect or control of one's temper, which are clearly private, the problems of medical ethics thrive in the overlap between these two areas of morality. Patients often claim control over their medical care on the grounds that their decisions are private, yet the very privacy of those decisions is protected by the medical profession's practice of confidentiality and by government regulation. The conflict between public and private morality is a key ingredient in many of the cases in this book.

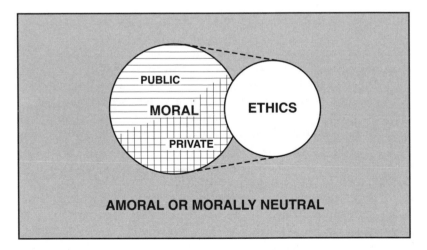

Figure 18-3

The tension between public and private morality arises between two sides of morality, not between the moral and the non-moral (Fig. 18–4). Abortion is a good example of a borderline issue. One may argue against abortion both as a private choice and as public policy, or one may argue that abortion has positive value as a private choice and should be tolerated or even encouraged as public policy. One may also take a mixed position, arguing against abortion as a private choice, but in favor of toleration as public policy or even in favor of funding it for the poor as a matter of justice. Both the public and private sides of these positions are moral stances that have ethical theory in the background.

One needs, therefore, to develop an ethical theory that provides for a reasonable relationship between public and private concerns. Therefore, as we discuss ethical theories in the following sections, we will describe how they deal with the tensions between public and private morality. The ability of an ethical theory to deal with this issue is one important measure of its success.

Distinguishing Good from Bad Morality

The most important measure of the success of an ethical theory, however, is its ability to distinguish the morally good or right from the morally bad or wrong. As one would expect, drawing this distinction is a matter of intense philosophical argument.

Since the early part of the nineteenth century, ethics has been dominated by two approaches; one distinguishes the good from the bad, the other the right

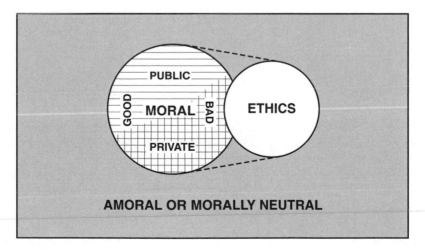

Figure 18-4

from the wrong. Utilitarianism, developed by Jeremy Bentham and John Stuart Mill, judges the moral goodness of actions by their consequences, especially the happiness they generate. Theories of rights and duties (often called deontological theories), developed under the inspiration of Immanuel Kant, hold that adherence to duty is the primary measure of moral rightness. Both are "single-key" theories because they argue that there is one fundamental test of the moral value of any course of action. Both theories work to apply their distinctive rule to what should be done in given situations. These single-key theories focus on the actions of individuals. They try to answer the question, "What should I do?" The next section of this chapter deals with the most prominent of these substantive theories.

Two subsequent sections deal with some recent developments in the discussion of ethical medicine. One deals with the emergence of autonomy as the dominant moral value in decision making, which, as we see it, transforms the question from *what* should be done to *who* should decide. The other discusses the approaches of a group of thinkers who are skeptical of the abstractions offered by philosophers who claim to answer the "what should be done" question. They variously appeal to the virtues or personal qualities of those who make decisions or to the processes of case-by-case analysis. In conclusion, we argue that all these ingredients are important for sound thinking about difficult medical ethical issues, and that it is not *what* someone decides nor *who* decides but how the decision is made that determines its morality.

What Should I Do?

Utilitarianism

Utilitarianism was developed by a group of late eighteenth- and nineteenth-century British philosophers. In the classic phrase of John Stuart Mill, a nineteenth-century philosopher and social reformer, a utilitarian considers those acts to be right that "produce the greatest happiness for the greatest number." Utilitarianism is a major root for the value of beneficence in medical ethics. Although there are many variations on this theme, utilitarian theories have certain common characteristics.

First, they are consequentialist, which means that they measure the goodness of an action by the value of its consequences, what happens as a result of the action. Since all actions have both good and bad consequences, it is more precise to say that utilitarianism is a theory of proportionality, meaning that the best action has the highest proportion of good to bad consequences. Cost-benefit analysis and other tools of contemporary economics and management have evolved from utilitarian thinking. Many medical decisions also use cost-benefit analysis. In a medical situation, the costs are not simply monetary but include psychological, social, and physical effects.

Second, utilitarian theories define right actions as those that produce a good that the theory specifies. Determining the proportion between good and bad consequences requires some notion of what good consequences are. Utilitarian theorists all develop such a concept, whether it be Jeremy Bentham's narrow concept of pleasure, happiness (which the Greeks called eudaimonia), or more contemporary views about quality of life. Right actions, in the utilitarian view, are those that produce more good in proportion to bad than any alternative.

Utilitarianism has the advantage of somehow feeling right. Pain and unhappiness are surely not good things and should be minimized, while pleasure, happiness, love, joy, and fulfillment are good things. Most people feel that good actions should produce happiness, not misery.

Moreover, utilitarianism promises to decide moral issues rationally. It is satisfying to add up the good consequences of an action on one side and the bad on another to arrive at a rational choice. Much modern decision theory and analysis of medical therapy, not to mention common sense, are based on such an approach. Utilitarianism tries to develop a clear bottom line for good decisions.

Carrying out the utilitarian program, however, turns out to be a complicated business. As medical situations shift and change, both costs and benefits are hard to predict. Utilitarians deal with such uncertainty by adding a factor of risk, probability, or chance to their calculations, comparing the probability of good outcomes with that of possible bad outcomes. For example, the utilitarian compares the risk of costly medical care and bad outcome to the chance of moderately expensive medical care and good outcome, the risks of physical and psychosocial costs to patient and family to the pleasures and benefits of each. A probability factor may be assigned to each of the more common complications of treatment. A negative or positive value can thus be assigned to each proposed course of action.

When we first encounter utilitarianism, the kind of thinking it requires seems straightforward and commonsensical. It seems to be the same kind of thinking we might use to decide which of three or four apartments to rent or which car to buy. As we try to analyze cases using utilitarian calculations, however, the work becomes increasingly difficult, more like weighing risks involved in various national defense strategies than common practical decisions. Because even simple decisions have innumerable possible consequences, ordinary choices can take on an overwhelming complexity. Utilitarianism is not as easy to apply as might at first appear.

Since utilitarianism focuses on results or consequences, such theories are the target of the traditional challenge, "Does the end justify the means?" The utilitarian argues that, if the result of two different actions is the same, the actions and their morality are the same. From a utilitarian perspective, the ends arrived at are precisely what justify whatever means are used. If a utilitarian concludes that it is best for a patient to die, distinctions among the means, for example between killing and letting die, become unimportant. In discussions of euthanasia, the utilitarian argues that the difference between killing a patient and letting the patient die is mainly the terrible costs in pain and suffering for both patient and family that letting die often involves.

Finally, the utilitarian does not limit the calculation of costs and benefits to those of the patient. While the principal costs and benefits may be the patient's, there are always others to be considered: family, other caretakers, the medical care system, and society as a whole. If utilitarianism insists that we act for the benefit of the greatest number, we must include all, even future generations, as factors in our calculations.

Taking the social context into account is both the greatest strength and the greatest weakness of utilitarianism. The theory recognizes that the public and the private spheres are closely connected and that individual decisions have wide-ranging social consequences. There was a day when health care decisions were strictly between physician and patient, but such simplicity no longer applies. Many areas of medicine are not as private as they used to be. Utilitarians argue that good decisions must take account of the consequences for families, the medical care system, employers, insurance companies, the government—in short, the whole society. The willingness of utilitarianism to take account of these factors, however, gives rise to one of the classic objections to the theory.

Utilitarianism sometimes seems to demand that we sacrifice some good, perhaps even the life, of an individual because that person's life is too "expensive" to other people. If a person's life is some, but only a small, benefit to himself and a great burden to others, the greatest happiness of the greatest number will be secured by sacrificing the individual. If terrorists, for example, demand that a government official be killed or they will use a nuclear bomb to destroy a major city, the utilitarian seems compelled to sacrifice one to save many. If very premature babies are destined to lead only a marginal life while making their parents' lives miserable and placing a great burden on society then, by utilitarian theory, it is best to insure that they die.

Some utilitarians have tried to deal with such violations of customary morality by developing a variation called "rule" utilitarianism. (Whether rule utilitarianism is a genuinely distinct theory or just a long-range version of the original or "act" utilitarian theory is a controversial question among philosophers.) Rule utilitarians argue that we should not judge individual actions but rather social rules, institutions, or practices. There are immediate benefits of giving in to terrorists, but the costs of the social practice of appeasement might easily outweigh them. The reverse may be said of the care of individuals. While an individual's care, viewed as a series of isolated acts, might be too expensive, the practice of providing costly care for the handicapped might provide an overall benefit to society.

Rule utilitarianism thus takes account of other moral traditions, notably that of individual rights. It can argue that the notion of rights that is central to many ethical arguments is only a quick way of expressing good social practices. The right to free speech, for example, is well justified by its results in opening communication in society and enhancing individual satisfaction. The utilitarian, however, argues that rights are not absolutes but are limited in situations in which honoring them would produce harmful consequences. The standard example is that the right of free speech does not protect someone who falsely cries "Fire!" in a crowded theater. Individual rights, the utilitarian claims, are social practices that are beneficial in the long run.

Several of our cases turn on a conflict between a benefit for the individual or society and some standard notion of rights or duties that seems to prohibit obtaining the benefit, or at least obtaining it in a certain way. In thinking about euthanasia, for example, the utilitarian compares the poor quality of a patient's life with the great costs of keeping him alive. Utilitarians interpret the discussion of the rights of a patient or spouse to make a decision, or about the duties of physicians, as merely ways of discussing the consequences of active euthanasia. They argue that their way of thinking about the issue, their ethical theory, is clearer and keeps our attention where it should be, on the good and bad consequences of each proposed course of action.

Whether one uses act or rule utilitarianism, however, the question remains: can the approach overcome the objection that it sacrifices individuals and their integrity to some wider good? The utilitarian takes individual rights to be no more than instruments of social benefit and individual integrity to be merely a means of producing good. For unmixed utilitarians there is finally no question but that individuals, whether themselves or others, should be sacrificed for the good of the whole. Recognizing this objection, most current forms of utilitarianism introduce some additional principles to dilute the impact of the theory on individuals.

Classical utilitarians, however, can deal with this objection by claiming that some of our moral intuitions are faulty and should be reconstituted in a utilitarian fashion. After all, the function of an ethical theory is to organize and systematize our morality. All of our present moral beliefs should not come through the process unchanged. Utilitarians can also point out that their theory at least accords with one of our basic intuitions about morality: that it should lead to human happiness. Rights and duties, they may claim, are not moral absolutes but make sense only when placed in the service of happiness.

While agreeing with the utilitarian that human well-being and fulfillment are crucial to morality, we part from the claim that the concept of human happiness can be developed sufficiently to provide a moral "bottom line" or single standard against which the goodness of actions can be measured. The notion of good or happiness is too rich and multifaceted to provide such a standard. Some people cling to lives that very few would consider worth living, while others who seem to live full and satisfying lives reject them with self-destructive behavior. The term "quality of life" has a nice ring, but it becomes entirely too vague when people try to apply it in individual situations. It does not seem possible to develop a sufficiently defined and acceptable notion of good, benefit, or best interest to allow someone to evaluate consequences as utilitarianism demands.

Even if there were a precise way to define happiness, working with utilitarian calculations would be a nightmare. Because every action has endless consequences, calculating the costs and benefits of alternative possibilities becomes a herculean task. Introducing risk further complicates the calculations. Several cases in this book, e.g. Christie, the Castelli Baby, Maggie, and Ed Martinez, show the difficulty of predicting outcome, especially when one tries to take account of improvements that might be brought about by new therapies. When, for example, the statistics for the survival of very premature newborns are constantly changing and the lives or deaths of the treated and the untreated are so unpredictably diverse, how does the utilitarian calculate whether or not to treat? This objection gains strength from the promise of utilitarianism to give definite "bottom-line" answers, to tell us the right thing to do.

Finally, the utilitarian claim that happiness or fulfillment is the ultimate value against which any other value can be measured fails to give adequate importance to staples of our moral thinking such as rights and personal integrity. As existentialists and others have observed, freedom and its accompanying responsibility do not always make people happy, but they are still part of our human dignity. Utilitarianism is too ready to see individuals, their rights, and their integrity merely as means to happiness without an inherent value of their own.

These objections to utilitarianism are neither original nor, as we have stated them, fatal to the theory. Their force, however, is to make the theory less obvious. These objections count against utilitarianism as an ethical theory, that is, against a way of thinking about morality. We are not criticizing it for giving the wrong results, much less criticizing those who hold the theory. But, at least taken by itself, we think it is an inadequate way to think about moral issues.

As we move beyond utilitarian theory, however, it will be well to take along the utilitarian's concern for human happiness and well-being. Some of the theories we are about to examine are so concerned with other aspects of morality that they neglect this essential element. We agree with the utilitarians that happiness and fulfillment must be part of our moral system; we only reject the consequentialist way utilitarians incorporate these realities in their theory.

The objections to utilitarianism naturally turn us to an ethics of duty. Typical theories of duty pay a great deal of attention to the integrity and importance of the individual and, since they do not rest their moral evaluation on consequences, they do not get snarled in the objectionable calculations of utilitarianism.

The Theory of Duties

Contemporary theories of duty take their inspiration from the work of Immanuel Kant, a philosopher of the late eighteenth century. Like utilitarianism, Kant's theory proposes a single rule for judging an action, but Kant proposes a rule of right action that he applies not to outcomes but to intentions, an aspect of morality that utilitarians say little about.

One of the principal objections to utilitarianism turns on the difficulties of calculating the consequences of our decisions. As our cases make clear, no one has full control of the outcome, even with good medical practice. Many consequences of our actions depend on chance, luck, or other factors outside our control. Because we only praise or blame people in a moral way for what they deliberately do, Kant argues that moral evaluation has to apply to something under our control. Kant therefore proposes that moral evaluation applies directly to the decision, to the decision-making act of the will, and not to consequences. As he puts it, "Nothing in the world—indeed nothing even beyond the world—can possibly be conceived which could be called good without qualification except a good will." Instead of looking at the consequences of actions, Kant focuses moral evaluation on the choice itself.

Kant calls the rule for judging good rules of action the "categorical imperative." Although he phrased it in several ways, the clearest expression of the categorical imperative for our purposes is, "Act so that you treat humanity, both in your own person and in that of another, always as an end and never merely as a means." Contemporary philosophers often refer to this as the respect principle, the principle that demands human respect for other people and for ourselves. The respect that health care professionals owe their patients is a special case of the respect that every person owes every other. Kantian ethics is the primary source for the principle of medical ethics that respect for each person means respecting their autonomous decisions.

Informed consent is a good example of the application of the respect principle. We have a duty to treat patients only with their consent because we have a moral obligation to respect their choices and free decisions. Obtaining consent treats patients as human beings, as people who exert control over their own lives, and not merely as objects or means to some purposes of ours.

People have what Kant calls "autonomy," the ability to make rules for themselves. Several cases in this book, notably Jill's, which discussed physician-assisted suicide, focus on the issues involved in autonomy. In contrast with act utilitarianism, the Kantian does not think it critically important whether people are happier for being told of the side effects of their drugs or their risk of being victims of genetically transmitted disease. The theory of moral duty holds that people should be told such things as part of the respect that doctors and nurses owe their patients.

Kant argues that the respect principle is morally valid because it can be universally or categorically applied. If you do not want to be treated without your consent, lied to about your medical care, or treated as a child or an incompetent, you should not treat others that way. As the golden rule has it, treat others as you would be treated. Kant argues that it makes no sense to want to be treated in a paternalistic, condescending, or not-fully-human way, that it is virtually self-contradictory to say "lie to me." Furthermore, there is no justification for treating people in similar circumstances differently from one another. The Kantian perspective in medical ethics, therefore, has strongly criticized paternalism and benevolent lying while emphasizing truth telling, autonomy, and informed consent.

Kant's moral theory is deontological (derived from the Greek word for "what one must do") because it uses the categorical imperative to develop a list of moral duties. The most general duties are binding on all human beings at all times.

Duties may be divided into positive duties and negative duties. Treating people with respect, for example, means at least that we should not lie to them. Not lying or not killing, therefore, are universal negative duties. In the tradition of Hippocratic medicine, the first and negative duty of physicians is to do no harm. On this theory, the negative duty, expressed in the biblical command as "Thou shalt not kill," is more fundamental and absolute than the obligation to give aid.

Positive duties, on the other hand, commit us to acting in certain ways. Positive obligations may be generated by explicit commitments, promises, or contracts or generated implicitly by social roles or customs. In an ethics of duty, physicians have a strong positive duty to patients they have accepted into their practices that is much stronger than to sick people in general. Nurses have similarly strong obligations to patients in a hospital for which they work. Hospitals also have special obligations to their patients and the local communities they serve.

Two examples illustrate the difference between positive and negative duties: the distinction between truth telling and lying and that between killing and letting die. Theories of moral duty hold that there is a very strong duty not to lie, but the positive duty to tell the truth is not as strong. In medical situations the duty to tell the truth is relative to many things, including the patient's level of understanding, physical and emotional condition, and desire to know. Cancer patients who ask pointed questions, for example, should be told the truth. Although there is a strong duty not to lie, the duty to tell the truth to those who do not seek it out, or who try to avoid it, is much weaker.

The distinction between positive and negative duties is also significant for its close connection to the distinction between killing and letting die, between active and passive euthanasia. Negative duties, since they are universally binding, have priority over positive ones. While not all theories of moral duty prohibit killing in every circumstance, they do recognize a substantial difference between killing and leveling off or reducing the level of medical care even while anticipating the patient's death. The positive obligation to provide medical care is relative to the technology available, the patient's condition and wishes, and the patient's relation to family and society. Although the duty to provide a certain level of medical care may depend on the circumstances, the duty not to kill is negative, definite, and much stronger; some even argue it is absolute.

Although it is part of the natural law rather than the Kantian tradition, the principle of double effect is another way to work out the implications of the distinction between positive and negative duties.

> In such [conflict] situations the evil caused as one goes about doing good has been viewed as justified or tolerable under a fourfold condition. (1) The action is good or indifferent in itself; it is not morally evil. (2) The intention of the agent is upright, that is, the evil effect is sincerely not intended. (3) The evil effect must be equally immediate causally with the good effect, for otherwise it would be a means to the good effect and would be intended. (4) There must be a proportionally grave reason for allowing the evil to occur.
> Richard A. McCormick, S.J., *Ambiguity in Moral Choice* (Milwaukee: Marquette University Press, 1973), page 1

Applied to pain relief for terminally ill patients, for example, the principle of double effect permits the morally neutral administration of morphine so long as the physician does not intend to hasten the patient's death and so long as giving morphine has both the good effect of relieving pain and the bad one of suppressing respiration. On the natural law account of moral action, double effect shows how the imperfect obligation to relieve pain can be compatible with the perfect obligation not to kill.

Of course, theories of moral duty do not find every instance of letting die to be morally acceptable. The fact that not treating is not doing something, an omission rather than a commission, is irrelevant when there is a clear and positive duty to act. Standing aside and letting salvageable patients die, as was sometimes done in the "Baby Doe" cases, is, on Kantian grounds, an inexcusable neglect of one's positive duties, not a morally acceptable "letting die." Among duty theorists, some would limit the duty to treat by the duty to honor the patient's wishes or those of the family, while others would limit these duties by distinguishing between ordinary and extraordinary care. Ordinary care, in this view, is the level of care demanded by the duty to respect another human being. Extraordinary care is in some way optional for the patient or is beyond that which we are strictly obliged to provide.

Codes of professional morality typically list the positive duties of health care providers. The American Nurses Association's Code for Nurses and the American Medical Association's Principles of Medical Ethics are two examples. Both begin by requiring practitioners to respect the human dignity of their patients (physicians) or clients (nurses). They then spell out what respect entails. Each of the codes requires that the patients' confidentiality be honored and that practitioners act to insure the integrity of medical care by taking action in cases of incompetent or unethical practice.

The standard codes of professional morality and our conventional ideas of duty are, however, only indirectly related to the fundamental duty of human respect. When one gets down to cases, matters become difficult. First, the obligations listed in the codes of nursing or medical practice sometimes conflict. The duty to respect a client's confidences, for example, can conflict with the duty to take action against incompetent or unethical practice.

Moreover, our obligations are not usually precisely defined. No one is opposed to respecting human dignity as long as what that means is left unspecified. When discussing voluntary euthanasia, however, some people hold that the practice respects the dignity of the patient by following the patient's wishes, while others argue that it destroys the dignity of health care professionals and undermines each person's duty to respect his or her own life.

An ethics of moral duty has several important strengths. First, grounding the respect principle with a golden rule argument is a very effective strategy. Second, the main duties of physicians and nurses, which are derived from the basic principle, are consonant with our fundamental moral intuitions, at least in their abstract expression. The problem with the theory of moral duties arises in the course of developing concrete moral guidance from the basic principle. In the abstract the theory has much to be said for it, but getting it to work for individual decisions raises some serious problems.

Before isolating the elements of a duty theory of morality that we want to retain, however, it will be useful to sketch out a related theory—the theory of moral rights.

Moral Rights
The theory of duties and the theory of moral rights are usually thought of as two sides of the same coin. If one person has a right to something, someone

else has the duty to deliver it, and any duties one might have generate corresponding rights in other people. If a physician accepts a patient into her practice, the patient has a right to that doctor's competent medical care. Likewise, the rights of patients generate duties. If patients have the right to know what is in their medical records, physicians or nurses in possession of the records have a duty to disclose the information. While rights and duties are correlative, there is a great philosophical controversy about which one is primary. Some philosophers hold that rights generate duties; others insist that it goes the other way around. Generally, philosophers who begin from a social or political perspective tend to make rights primary, while those who start from the perspective of individual decisions tend to take duties as fundamental.

As shown in the previous section, starting from duties has the philosophical advantage of resting on a strong argument. Beginning with rights, on the other hand, provides a position with great rhetorical power. As one contemporary philosopher has phrased it, rights are "trump cards" that, when played, settle the issue in favor of the one playing them. People love having rights, and the more of them the better. No one can have too many of them. The same can hardly be said of duties; even one duty sometimes seems too many. The founding documents of the United States are couched in terms of rights, dependent as they are on the thinking of natural rights theorists of the eighteenth century such as John Locke and Jean-Jacques Rousseau. In the words of the Declaration of Independence, "We hold these truths to be self-evident, that all men are created equal; that they are endowed by their Creator with certain inalienable rights; that among these are life, liberty, and the pursuit of happiness." This single sentence contains all the important elements of a theory of rights, and each element shows both the advantages and disadvantages of such a theory.

The first element of any theory of rights is the scope of the theory: who has the rights? The Declaration speaks of "all men," which in its historical context meant something close to "white, male property owners." In the U.S. Constitution, each slave was counted as three-fifths of a person in determining the population of the states. The document assumes that women would not vote; it does not challenge the laws in various states limiting the right to vote to property owners or imposing a tax or religious test on voting. Such measures substantially restricted the scope of constitutional rights until well into this century.

In contemporary terms, the conflict over abortion and some cases of euthanasia is a conflict over the scope of rights. In *Roe v. Wade*, the Supreme Court held that, since the issue was so variously debated by philosophers and theologians, no one can be sure that fetuses incapable of surviving outside the womb are really persons. Since only persons have constitutional rights, fetuses could not be said to have such rights during the first two trimesters of their mothers' pregnancy. The Supreme Court went on to rule that, because fetuses fell outside the scope of full human rights, abortion during the first two trimesters was a private right of women that could not be prohibited by state or federal law.

The second element of a theory of rights is the source or origin of the rights. The framers of the U.S. Constitution held that God gave people rights. The theological argument is widely criticized today by both believers and nonbelievers. Many Christians point out that biblical ethics says more about duties or God's love than it does about rights. Religious people from other traditions observe that the theory of rights is not part of their heritage, while nonbelievers observe that attempting to ground rights on a religious basis compromises the theory in a secular, pluralist society.

Some contemporary theories of rights claim a basis in moral intuitions, while others derive rights from some version of the respect principle, but the most prominent recent efforts derive rights from some version of a social contract. Deriving rights from the respect principle subordinates them to duties instead of giving them a primary role in morality. If rights discourse becomes derivative, it loses much of its rhetorical punch. Moreover, if rights are derived from duties and we need to rank them in order of importance, we will find rights just as vague and conflicted as duties.

Deriving rights from a social contract seems to offer a way of establishing them rationally on the basis of some impulse or structure shared by all. If all humans are fundamentally self-interested, for example, we would all rationally agree on rules that allowed each of us to maximize our self-interest. On the other hand, if all humans accept some principle of mutual respect, then we would establish a social system of respect. Social contract theorists, however, disagree about the nature of those who enter into the contract and about the implications of the contract for the societies in which we now live. Thus, they tend to undermine their own attempts at rational justification.

The list of rights is the third element of any rights theory. The Declaration of Independence does not claim to list all rights but only certain among them. The thinking of the Supreme Court in defining a constitutional right to privacy is a good example of how complex rights arguments can become. In a famous case striking down a Connecticut law that forbade the sale of contraceptives in the state (*Griswold v. Connecticut*), the Supreme Court found a right to privacy in the "penumbra," literally the shadows, of the Fourteenth Amendment.

The list of rights asserted in medical situations, like the duties of health care providers, has been shifting and difficult to define. Some have held that there is a right to die or a right to die with dignity. There are also controversial claims about the right to medical care. For example, who would have the duty to provide the medical care demanded by those exercising the right?

Some of the conflicts about rights can be resolved by making a distinction between claim rights and liberties, a distinction very similar to that between positive and negative duties. Liberties guarantee the freedom of people to act as they please, while claim rights give people claims on others. The right to vote, for example, is a claim right because the citizen who is entitled to vote has a claim against election judges and polling place workers to make voting possible. Welfare rights are also claim rights, since the government has granted poor people the right to claim certain benefits. Such a claim to benefits is commonly called an entitlement. Most of the rights guaranteed in the basic documents of the United States, however, are liberties. Free speech, for example, is the right not to be interfered with in the expression of one's opinion, but it does not commit the government or anyone else to providing newspaper space or another forum for the expression of opinion.

Whether the rights under discussion are liberties or claim rights is often unclear in a medical context. Some people take the right to die to mean the right to refuse medical treatment, an assertion of the liberty to be left alone. Others believe that the right to die means that patients in certain circumstances have the right to medical help in easing their death or committing suicide. Sometimes the right to medical care means no more than that medical care should be provided without discrimination with regard to religion, race, sex, or national origin. Others argue that there is a positive or claim right to a certain level of medical care. They argue that everyone has a right to medical attention and a claim against society to obtain it.

The rights of the handicapped are typical of the complexity of the issue. Some advocates for the handicapped argue that the rights of the handicapped are liberties that individual handicapped people may or may not exercise. They take the right to treatment to be a liberty that one could exercise or not as one judged best, similar, perhaps, to freedom of speech. Others argue that the handicapped have claims against society to insure their life is protected. They claim that handicapped newborns, for example, have positive rights to treatment such that not treating violates their rights. In some instances, the right to treatment is so strong a claim that denying the right may be morally unacceptable. Newborns with severe but easily remedied problems, for example, have a right to treatment even though their parents, perhaps for religious reasons, do not wish to exercise that right or a hospital, facing an unpaid bill, does not wish to provide it. The children's rights, in these cases, compel treatment even over some legitimate objections.

In a far larger number of cases, however, the right to treatment is less compelling. In these cases the question shifts from what rights require to the right to decide. Instead of asking what we should do, we ask who should decide. In terms of the moral issues that arise in medicine, should patients, relatives, physicians, or society say what should be done? The discussion of who should decide arises from the theory of moral rights and has become so important in medical ethics that it needs developed treatment.

Who Should Decide?

The Patient

The currently dominant view is that patients should decide about their own medical care. As the title of the play put it, Whose life is it anyway? There is a very broad consensus on this point that accords with the moral theories we have already discussed. Theories of rights hold that a person has a right to decide about his or her own medical care. Even those who make odd or unintelligent decisions nonetheless have the right to make them. Moreover, physicians and nurses have a duty to help people make their own decisions, to respect these autonomous decisions, and to help carry them out. Furthermore, there are utilitarian grounds for respecting autonomous decisions since they are likely to produce the greatest happiness for the people most involved.

Both morality and the law recognize the fundamental value of informed consent—the right of individuals, after they are sufficiently informed of their options, to consent to or even direct their own medical care. Patients have both a constitutional and common law right to physical integrity. The Supreme Court, in its 1990 decision in *Cruzan v. Director, Missouri Department of Health* reviewed a number of previous decisions and ended by declaring:

> As these cases demonstrate, the common-law doctrine of informed consent is viewed as generally encompassing the right of a competent individual to refuse medical treatment. . . . [F]or purposes of this case, we assume the United States Constitution would grant a competent person a constitutionally protected right to refuse lifesaving hydration and nutrition.

There is a legal consensus that the health-care decisions of conscious, rational adults are matters of personal liberty. As long as they do not press their views or their care on others, society is content to leave people alone.

Extending Autonomy: Advance Directives and Surrogate Decisions

The difficult cases, however, concern the care of patients who, to some degree, lack consciousness, competence, or maturity. People who are ill are almost always compromised in one or more of these dimensions. Illness involves some loss of control. When patients are unable to decide for themselves, who is to make decisions for them?

Advance directives allow patients to extend their liberty by refusing medical treatment when they cannot express their wishes directly. Several types of advance directives are in common use.

Do Not Resuscitate.   Hospitalized patients may refuse cardiopulmonary re-suscitation, and physicians commonly enter such Do Not Resuscitate (DNR) orders in patient's charts. Communities are working to make DNR orders effective in nursing homes and other out-of-hospital settings.

Living Will.   Living wills are the most widely known form of advance direc-tive. All states now recognize some form of living will, but the specific provi-sions vary. As a tool for extending the range of a patient's autonomous choices, the living will is of limited use. The wording in most states confines its application to those who are clearly dying and limits the therapies that can be removed under its provisions.

Specific Medical Directives.   Patients can, after reviewing a number of sce-narios and treatment alternatives, negotiate care plans with their physicians. The scenarios illustrate various situations of patient incapacity along with the prognosis associated with alternative treatments. Patients can choose in ad-vance what they would want in each situation. This is the most individualized form of advance directive, but there are not yet many reports of its effective use.

Durable Power of Attorney for Health Care.   All states allow individuals to execute a durable power of attorney for health care, a legal document giv-ing specific powers to a personal representative. The representative represents someone's wishes when the patient is permanently or temporarily unable to present them directly. This is a very flexible tool because the power of attor-ney can be as general or specific, restricted or broad, as an individual desires. Unless the representative has a good knowledge of the patient's wishes and the courage to express them to caregivers, however, the device will not serve to carry out the patient's intentions.

There are many important situations in which it is not possible to represent the patient's own judgment. Infants, young children, the mentally handicapped, and many others either never could or never have made any decisions about their own medical care. When decisions must be made for them, a surrogate must act on their behalf. Traditional morality grants parents, spouses, or other relatives the right to make decisions for such patients. Much contemporary ethical theory, with its emphasis on autonomy, has difficulty justifying or ra-tionalizing this tradition.

One justification for this power to make decisions is that relatives are most likely to know and act in a family member's best interest. For example, young children should eat their vegetables and drink their milk because parents know what is good for them. Although this justification is usually valid, superior knowledge may not entirely justify a relative's decision about life or death care. Even very bright and well-educated parents, for example, do not have the knowledge required to make decisions about the medical treatment of their child in an intensive care nursery.

Perhaps parents, spouses, or other relatives are the right ones to make these decisions for their children, not because they have superior knowledge, but because they are the ones most concerned and involved with their loved one's care. In contrast to the previous argument, which rests on knowledge of what makes a good life, this argument is based on the duties of family membership. While the assumption is generally valid, some of the unusual cases that arise in medicine challenge it. Not all parents are models of care and concern for their children. Parents who are suddenly faced with raising a handicapped child or relatives responsible for a severely damaged adult are immersed in a terrible conflict, even what might be termed a "conflict of interest." They may want to do the right thing for the patient, but they also want to do what is best for themselves and perhaps for other members of the family. There is a tragic conflict here and, without trying to assign any blame, we cannot automatically assume that parents or relatives are acting out of wholehearted concern for the patient.

The relation between knowledge and concern seems to be circular. We cannot know whether, for example, parents are adequately concerned for their child if we do not know what they should do, yet only because we do not know what to do have we turned to parental concern as our standard of judgment. If the substituted judgment of parents is difficult to justify, the cases of husbands, wives, and other relatives is even harder. Do spouses have a moral duty to tear their lives completely apart to care for one another? How far do such duties go, and how do they interact with other duties someone might have? When there is no spouse, how does one decide among the wishes, concerns, and conflicts of children and other relatives?

Providing an ethical justification for the right of kin to make decisions for one another is difficult both in theory and in practice. Suppose spouses have been at odds in recent months, even thinking seriously about divorce? Suppose, as happens often enough, that the adult children argue fiercely about the kind and amount of medical care that is appropriate for a critically ill parent; who are the relevant kin to make decisions in such situations?

The inability of relatives to make decisions is sometimes in conflict with the medical necessity that decisions be made. In such situations, physicians or nurses frequently become involved in decision-making.

Doctors and Nurses

Robert Veatch introduced the phrase "generalization of expertise" to characterize the tendency of physicians to move from what he terms their legitimate area of medical expertise to assume the status of moral experts. He speaks of physicians acting as a kind of priesthood when they make decisions for others. The view that physicians and nurses should stay within their medical and technical expertise and not venture into the sphere of moral decision-making is widely held in the medical ethics community. Philosophers are wary of paternalism, of interfering with someone's choices for that person's own good.

Physicians and nurses, however, are often drawn into making decisions for patients. Sometimes they act because the patient is unable to function autonomously and there is no cohesive or responsible family to act for the patient. On other occasions nurses and physicians influence decisions because they have a better knowledge of the patient's needs or interests. Because they know other patients and the general course of a given disease, they are often in a better position than the patients or families to make judgments. While not all of these examples are strictly paternalistic, they are examples of the way caregivers move beyond the narrowly medical and become deeply involved in moral and human decisions.

Physicians or nurses are also involved in decisions by the way they present information or bring up questions. There is a good chance that the way information is conveyed, the values and the biases that inevitably accompany any presentation, will have a powerful impact on the decision. Nurses are often closer than physicians to patients and family, especially in critical care situations when the physicians involved are not the primary care doctors with whom patients and family are comfortable. Physicians will often ask nurses to find out what the family wants or even to guide family discussions so that necessary decisions can be made. Neither physicians nor nurses are morally neutral, and it is difficult to see how they could be.

In less technically sophisticated and more stable times, the health care professional was usually the family doctor working in the community hospital. He usually knew the patient and the family, often sharing their background and values. In these circumstances it was far easier for the physician to arrive at decisions that were congruent with those of patient and family. Now it is more commonly the case that physicians and nurses are taking care of strangers. Health care providers should therefore be sensitive to the diversity of their patients' values and be reluctant to impose their own values on them.

Many philosophers, as part of their critique of paternalism, argue that physicians lack the moral standing to be involved in the moral aspects of decision-making, but the tradition of physicians, the law, and the general view of society expects them to be. The Hippocratic oath demands that physicians act for the benefit of their patients and, implicitly, to determine what that benefit is. As an aspect of licensing physicians and restricting drugs, the law makes physicians the exclusive gatekeepers to certain therapies. It also requires physicians to report cases of suspected child neglect or abuse as well as certain communicable diseases. Many people still expect their physicians to provide personal or moral guidance. None of these functions is simply technical; their gatekeeping role inevitably involves physicians in the moral lives of their patients. If a physician believes a patient is making a mistake about his or her medical care, that physician must try to persuade the patient of the error. Ultimately, the physician may acquiesce to the patient's decision, resign from the case, or seek legal intervention to order treatment. The role of physicians, as defined by themselves, the law, and society, demands that they not participate in what they regard as immoral decisions.

Several conclusions follow from the discussion thus far. One is that none of the single-key, rule-based theories provides a complete and satisfactory solution to the problems raised in contemporary medical ethics. In particular, rights theories lead us to consider who has the rights. When we think about who is called upon to make a particular decision, we are led to reflect on that person's character. In some cases, people who ordinarily have particular rights do not exercise them in ways that seem morally acceptable. We challenge selfish parents or greedy doctors because these qualities conflict with their social role. Considerations of social role and the character of individuals making decisions has led to a resurgence of interest in the ethics of moral character or, as it has come to be called, "virtue ethics."

Protests Against Abstract Theory

In the past ten years, biomedical ethics has developed an increased awareness of its own history and roots. Much of modern bioethics arose from religious concerns with issues of life and death in the context of increasingly effective medical technology. A long tradition of Roman Catholic and Jewish concern with these issues was followed by Protestant interest and finally by philosophers operating without any particular religious tie. Philosophers tended to view medical ethics as an exciting arena for the debate between utilitarian and deontological ethical theory. While they lacked the concern for the spiritual care of individual patients that motivated those who approached medical ethics from a religious perspective, philosophers often brought increased intellectual rigor to the discussion.

Concern with medical ethics reinvigorated philosophy. It seemed for a while that medicine had saved the life of ethics, rescuing it from completely abstract arguments about the right and the good, but philosophers soon returned to their love of abstractions. Several philosophical movements, however, arose to fight this tendency again. While quite diverse among themselves, theories of moral pluralism, virtue ethics, feminist ethics, and casuistry have all challenged the dominance of traditional ethical theories.

The emphasis in all of these challenges is on thinking about the moral issues that arise in medicine from an experiential or "bottom-up" perspective. Writers who emphasize moral diversity begin with skepticism about the ability of traditional moral theories to provide a coherent or persuasive account of the moral differences that mark modern cultures. They argue that peoples' morality arises from their particular culture, and that the dominant secular culture of American public life and politics provides only one of many views about medicine. They find philosophical proposals for a one-size-fits-all theory unconvincing. If this point is accepted, one must then work out a medical ethics in relation to one's own culture. The following accounts discuss some of the ways philosophers have worked on this diverse project.

Virtue Ethics

The virtue ethics movement is a loose-knit reaction against rationalist moral systems. Much of its theory is drawn from Aristotle, whose *Nicomachean Ethics* describes the character and habits of good men in his society. He hoped that such descriptions and a general discussion of what made men good would guide young men toward living noble lives.

Virtue ethics is of particular interest to those who see the medical profession as a moral community. Because it views physicians and nurses as moral agents with special commitments and responsibilities, virtue ethics invites consideration of the development of good doctors. It returns to the Socratic quest for ways of educating people to live and act well.

In the *Ethics,* Aristotle lays out an approach to virtue. He considers that each virtue regulates a human drive or feeling; virtue or human excellence consists in the proper control and direction of our drives. Courage, for example, controls fear and confidence. It is midway between opposing vices— cowardice, which is a deficiency, and rashness, which is an excess. The truly courageous man, Aristotle thought, dealt with his fear and acted effectively in conflict. He had enough aggressive drive to fight without running away, yet not so much that he put himself or others in senseless danger.

Aristotle describes many virtues in detail and also includes a lengthy discussion of friendship in the *Ethics.* He rarely mentions principles and offers no rules for right action. Although he has high praise for practical wisdom and considers it the most important virtue, he does not think that morality can be reduced to any single key.

If one takes an Aristotelian approach to morality, a good life is not a matter of living and dying by the rules. Patients—that is, all of us—need to live and die with dignity and courage. While "death with dignity" is in danger of becoming a cliché, Aristotelians are committed to describing the character of a dignified life and death.

From the viewpoint of virtue ethics, the moral character of physicians, nurses, and other caregivers is critical. They need to approach their work as a human enterprise in which they pursue both technical and personal excellence. The central virtues of health care providers are, according to Edmund Pellegrino, compassion, trustworthiness, wisdom, and personal integrity. No set of laws or regulations, no matter how vigorously enforced, can insure that people do the right thing. The Aristotelian insists that morally good deeds flow from virtuous people.

To those who approach moral issues looking for the right rule or decision procedure, virtue ethics seems evasive. The virtue ethics tradition rarely answers the question "What should I do?" It insists that we look to role models more than rules, and role models sometimes break rules or cut new life paths through societies overgrown with laws and regulations. Insofar as medical ethics has developed in an American climate in which the primary place for moral argument is courts of law, virtue ethics is bound to seem "soft" and indecisive.

Virtue ethics is also vulnerable to the charge of cultural relativism. Aristotle was too ready to accept the roles his society assigned to men and women, slaves and free people. An earlier generation of medical ethicists praised paternalistic physicians and passive nurses. An ethics of principles and rules sets standards by which to judge and possibly advance a culture. A virtue ethic has a tendency to enshrine the status quo.

But a complete picture of medical ethics requires a place for virtue. We all live in a complex web of social roles, and our lives and decisions cannot be taken out of these contexts. The case of Ms. Williams (Chapter 5) in this volume illustrates the importance of virtue in medical ethics. Furthermore, developing the moral character of physicians and nurses requires a fuller account of the good life than an ethic of rules can provide.

Feminist Medical Ethics

Feminist ethics is as diverse as feminism itself. There are feminists of every philosophical stripe, from utilitarian to deontologial, from libertarian to socialist. Admitting its insufficiency, we will limit the discussion here to virtue feminism.

It might appear ironic to discuss feminist ethics in the same breath as virtue ethics for Aristotle was no feminist. But much feminist thinking in medical ethics can be understood as employing Aristotle's methodology in a very different social and medical context. Feminists choose different hero(ines) than did Aristotle and propose a very different picture of the good life. Where Aristotle might endorse physicians that many contemporary people would criticize as authoritarian or paternalistic, feminists endorse caring physicians who develop a therapeutic partnership with their patients. While feminists would universally reject Aristotle's male-centered views, some begin as he does by surveying the possibilities and requirements for a good life. Both propose experiential approaches to ethics that try to keep it in contact with the way people actually live and choose. And both believe that morality must be deeply concerned with the character of individuals and the moral character of the society in which they live.

Much feminist medical ethics has been influenced by studies of moral development. Some of the first studies in this field of psychology dealt only with male subjects. When the studies were expanded to include female subjects, none of the females were found to be operating on what the experimenters defined as the highest level of moral cognitive development—acting according to principle for the sake of the principles themselves. This conclusion provoked a sharp reaction, especially from feminists. Several subsequent studies challenged the conclusion by arguing that women developed moral maturity along a different cognitive path. That path was less marked by distinct stages and more concerned with complex and particular situations. It was less concerned with abstract rules of correct action. (See the review article by Alisa Carse in the volume edited by Suzanne Gordon et al. and cited in "Suggestions for Further Reading," at the end of this chapter.)

Some feminist thinkers identify feminist ethics with an ethic of care. A care ethic is based on personal involvement with all the participants in a difficult moral situation. It is less concerned than an ethics of rules with making a uniquely correct decision, more concerned with sustaining relationships with all those involved. Care is seen as a personal quality of working through a moral situation while keeping human relationships as intact as possible.

As one would expect, those who believe a moral theory ought to deliver principled answers to the question of what an individual should do criticize an ethics of care. Many feminists criticize it for marking women with a stereotype—caregiver—from which many women have worked to escape. They protest that the meaning of a caregiver's life has often been determined by those to whom care is given, mostly men and children, rather than by the (usually female) caregivers themselves. Identifying caregiving as a moral ideal challenges the primacy of autonomy, especially the autonomy of women. An ethics of care, therefore, suffers from the general weaknesses of virtue ethics noted in the discussion of Aristotle's ethics. By arguing for the moral significance of care, this type of feminist ethics not only refuses to answer the "what should I do?" question that much traditional medical ethics wants answered, but also argues for a virtue that is at odds with the freedom and autonomy central to American secular culture.

Casuistry

Yet another critique of abstract and universalist ethical theories comes from those who advocate focusing on particular cases and answering "what to do" questions. These thinkers take their model from the practice of law. And legal reasoning, as one can see from the frequent references in this book's cases, is the source for much of the medical ethics discussion in the United States. This approach separates from virtue and feminist ethics in its dedication to providing answers to individual questions. The legal system, after all is said and done, hands down decisions. It differs from the theories presented earlier in this chapter in working case by case; it is often marked by skepticism about abstractions.

Among legal practitioners there is an ongoing debate about the proper role of judges and the limits of judicial power. One school holds that cases should be decided one at a time, with full respect for the facts of particular cases and detailed attention to precedent set by previous cases of a similar kind. When the case-by-case method appears in medical ethics, it is called "casuistry," and it is skeptical of attempts by judges or other decision-makers to use abstract moral theories. Lawyers and judges are rarely given to theorizing when there are decisions to be made and time is of the essence.

Because it is so opposed to abstract theorizing, casuistry is hard to discuss. Most of its advocates write about it by describing the history of certain developments in law that they regard as wholesome and beneficial, such as the court decision to remove Karen Ann Quinlan from a respirator.

There is an obvious difficulty in relying on legal precedent, the history of legal decisions in related cases. Once precedents are set in one direction, no matter how many people regard that direction as irrational, the law may seem condemned to follow the course for a long time. To this objection, philosophers add their concern about the casuists' abandonment of moral theory.

Casuists and theoreticians have probably overstated their differences. Many court decisions plainly draw their inspiration from moral theory. They are not innocent of philosophy. The emphasis on autonomy in contemporary America is supported both by moral theory and by a legal tradition directly connected to the U. S. Constitution. The founders who framed that document were greatly influenced by their reading of such philosophers as Jean-Jacques Rousseau and John Locke. Reflecting this synthesis, the final chapter takes the practical reasoning of law as an important ingredient in developing a way that theory and practice can work together.

Conclusion

We hope the conflicts among the theories that we have described do not leave you with a sense of frustration and failure. We agree that none of these theories provides a complete guide to good action, but we do not accept the pessimistic view that all arguments about morality are therefore futile. There is much to be learned from each of the theories discussed in this chapter, even if none is sufficient by itself. In the next chapter we will try to show how the moral theories we have been discussing can be fit together in a way that takes advantage of the strengths and minimizes the weaknesses of each.

Suggestions for Further Reading

There is much more to be said about the moral problems that arise in medicine and about the philosophical theories that deal with them. We hope the preceding pages have given you an appetite for more. Here are some accessible sources for further reading in medical ethics.

Many anthologies include articles in philosophy and in medical ethics. Some of the most widely available and complete are: Arras and Steinbock, *Ethical Issues in Modern Medicine*, Beauchamp and Walters, *Contemporary Issues in Bioethics*, Mappes and Degrazia, *Biomedical Ethics*, Munson, *Intervention and Reflection*, Kuhse and Singer, *Bioethics, an Anthology*, and Robinson, Berry, and McDonnell, *A Health Law Reader*.

Several contemporary treatments of ethical theory that repay the reader's serious attention, among them: John Rawls, *A Theory of Justice*, Smart and Williams, *Utilitarianism: For and Against*, Alasdair MacIntyre, *After Virtue*, and Alan Donagan, *The Theory of Morality*. The virtue ethics tradition is well represented in Pellegrino and Thomasma's *The Virtues in Medical Practice*, moral pluralism in Engelhardt's *The Foundations of Bioethics*, and casuistry in Jonsen's *The Birth of Bioethics*. The feminist tradition of care ethics is presented in Gordon et al., *Caregiving: Readings in Knowledge, Practice, Ethics, and Politics*. A number of fine books provide a unified view of the problems of medical ethics including Jonsen, Sigler, and Winslade, *Clinical Ethics*, and Beauchamp and Childress, *Principles of Biomedical Ethics*. In addition to further readings, each of these volumes provides useful references to still more of the work in the field.

The classics, available in numerous editions, always reward the reader: Aristotle, *Nicomachean Ethics*, Immanuel Kant, *Foundations of the Metaphysics of Morals*, and John Stuart Mill, *Utilitarianism*.

Current issues in medical ethics are discussed in the *Hastings Center Report* and *The Kennedy Institute of Ethics Journal*. In almost every issue, the *Journal of the American Medical Association (JAMA)* and the *New England Journal of Medicine* carry articles that discuss significant ethical issues. Since biomedical ethics is such a rapidly changing field, readers need periodicals to keep up.

This chapter was written as a primer in medical ethics, an outline of the basic vocabulary and ideas in the field. It is designed only to get you started. Our greatest hope is that it stimulates you to read further in the field.

chapter

19

✳ ✳ ✳ ✳ ✳

Making Moral Decisions:
A Process Approach

For most medical decisions, there is a professional and social consensus on what should be done and a relatively simple process for determining it. Benefits and costs are usually clear, duties are apparent, and the patient readily consents to the physician's proposal for treatment.

Tough decisions arise when costs are not clear, duties are not obvious, when the patient's desires are different from those of the medical team, or when the standard solutions are no longer appropriate. In such circumstances, when people do not know what should be done and it is not clear who should decide, we have found it helpful to think about how good decisions can be made, to think about the process rather than the product.

Conflict and tragedy raise medical and moral issues, but so do social and technological change. The historical accounts in this chapter show that neither medicine nor morality are fixed in stone. The standards of good medicine develop as new technology is introduced and as social values change. Ethics, our systematic thinking about morality, also changes with the time, culture, and circumstance; think how our attitudes to slavery and race have changed in 150 years. Ethical debate changes morality because new practices require new justification or criticism. Similarly morality, or what we do, may change ethics, or how we think about what we do. Practice may at times lead theory, just as at other times theory may guide practice. Thus ethics, morality, and medicine have a dynamic interaction.

This interaction can be seen in some of the changes that have occurred in medical practice in recent decades. Each of the following four events introduced important changes in how medicine is practiced and in how we think about those practices. In the course of discussing these landmarks, we will begin to explain how our approach to good decision making works.

Four Medical and Moral Landmarks

The Nuremberg Trials and Informed Consent

At the end of World War II, the trials of war criminals at Nuremberg brought to light the atrocities committed by Nazi Germany against Jews, Gypsies, and other "non-Aryan" people. Some of these atrocities involved drafting unwilling subjects into medical experiments. As part of the legal process of prosecuting Nazis for these crimes, the tribunal at Nuremberg enunciated principles against involuntary subjection to research:

> The voluntary consent of the human subject is essential. This means that the person involved should have legal capacity to give consent; should be so situated as to be able to exercise free power of choice, without the intervention of force, fraud, deceit, duress, overreaching or other ulterior form of constraint or coercion; and should have sufficient knowledge and comprehension of the subject matter involved as to enable him to make an understanding and enlightened decision.
> *Trials of War Criminals before the Nuremberg Military Tribunals*, 1948

Examination of the Nazi crimes gradually altered our thinking about consent in medical experiments, and also for everyday therapeutic procedures. What was implicit in medical practice for centuries was brought to the surface by these historic trials.

Response to the revelations at Nuremberg was slow. Even after the Declaration of Helsinki (a statement of the Eighteenth World Medical Assembly meeting in Helsinki, Finland, in 1964), which reaffirmed the moral rejection of experiments without adequate consent, many researchers did not see the connection between their work and the Nazi medical experiments. In Tuskegee, Alabama, for example, the U.S. Public Health Service continued its observation of untreated syphilis until news reporters broke the story in 1972, over 25 years after it was discovered that penicillin effectively treated the disease.

It was even more difficult for many in the medical community to connect the notion of informed consent with therapy. Many thought that, by virtue of presenting themselves for examination, patients implicitly gave doctors both a request for a diagnosis and an authorization of treatment. Physicians viewed fully informed consent either as a noisome distraction or as an ideal beyond the grasp of ordinary medical practice. Asking for consent after explaining all of the risks of complications and side effects seemed both excessively time consuming and opened the possibility of frightening patients away from clearly beneficial care.

Several cases in this book illustrate how difficult it is to inform patients or relatives of all the medical facts that are important in making good decisions.

For example, Maggie does not want to be put on "the darn machines." Does she mean she does not want to be resuscitated after a brief, medication-induced cardiac arrest? Can physicians obtain informed consent in advance for all possible contingencies? The case of Christie raises the issue whether bias is an inevitable side effect of giving information. How should physicians handle those cases for which refusing treatment is morally or legally intolerable? What are the limits of ethical persuasion, and when does laying out the facts become manipulation?

Physicians increasingly recognize that consent is not a single event, but, especially in the course of an extended illness with a number of treatment options at various stages, informed consent is an ideal, at best the product of a lengthy process involving the full moral personality of patients, families, physicians, nurses and other caregivers. The moral value of informed consent depends on the process of obtaining it.

The "Johns Hopkins" Baby

In the early 1970s a baby was born at the Johns Hopkins Hospital with Down syndrome and duodenal atresia, a blockage of the upper part of the intestine. Without surgery to open the obstruction, it would have been impossible to feed the baby. After lengthy consultation with senior physicians at the hospital who recommended the operation, the baby's parents decided to refuse their consent. The infant was placed in a back room on the ward and died the following week of starvation and dehydration.

At that time such decisions were not rare. There was no established view in the medical community about the treatment of newborns with Down syndrome, and there had been little public debate on the issue. A standard recommendation for many otherwise healthy Down syndrome infants was that they be institutionalized immediately so that the parents "would not become too attached to them." Community services and support for the mentally handicapped were minimal, and an entire life spent in an institution was the fate of many such children. Surgical treatment for such mentally impaired babies was considered optional because, without medical, educational, or social support, vigorous intervention was not a benefit to the children, much less to their families or society.

Thinking about care of the mentally handicapped was beginning to change, however. After considerable reflection and discussion, Dr. Robert Cooke, chairman of the Department of Pediatrics at Johns Hopkins, and officials from the Kennedy Foundation decided to recreate the drama of the decision in a film that was used as a starting point for a panel discussion on the ethics of treating children with Down syndrome. Challenging the assumptions underlying the original decision, members of the panel suggested new ways to help parents cope with their Down's children and encouraged the development of community support services. They criticized the practice of institutionalizing the mentally handicapped. They also challenged the exclusive right of parents to decide, arguing that either foster care or adoption were practical alternatives when parents were unable to cope with a handicapped child.

The political prominence of the Kennedy family and its commitment to helping the mentally handicapped also fostered social change. The Educational Rights of the Handicapped Act (1974) ultimately entitled each handicapped child to an individualized treatment plan in a public educational facility. Facilities for community living and work, although still inadequate, have generally replaced institutions for the mentally handicapped.

For a number of years after the publicity surrounding the "Hopkins Baby," when an infant with Down syndrome required surgery, discussions about the child's rights, the benefits of surgery or other treatment, and a multitude of moral considerations were held among the parents, physicians, and others involved in the case. A consensus gradually evolved. This common view of the prognosis and appropriate care of the mentally handicapped is now so strong that, when a Down syndrome child is born with an associated problem, the presentation to the parents consists mainly of explaining the need for and benefit of corrective procedures. Medicine informs and parents consent. The decision-making process no longer deals with all the ambiguity of individual decisions. (We agree with the President's Commission on Biomedical Ethics and the vast majority of commentators in medical ethics that the much publicized Baby Doe case in Bloomington, Indiana, was an unusual and unjustifiable exception to this consensus.) Failure to treat vigorously is now intolerable.

It is clear that the original decision at Johns Hopkins would be morally unacceptable today. What has changed? In the case of Down syndrome, the medical facts are similar, although we can better manage heart problems and infections in newborns. But the important changes are in the social attitudes that began with the professional and public debate that followed the film. Our moral sensitivity toward the mentally handicapped has become more acute, and we have become more willing to nurture and support them. As our moral view of the handicapped has changed, so have the boundaries of what is acceptable. Changes in morality have led to changes in medical practice.

Spina Bifida, Technology, and the Non-mentally Handicapped Infant

The attention initially focused on newborns with Down syndrome gradually spread to other handicapped infants, those with physical defects but no intellectual impairment. Children with spina bifida pose different questions about quality of life for the handicapped. In the 1950s few children with spina bifida were treated. The great risks of operating on the newborn and technical problems with shunts for hydrocephalus were major deterrents to intervention. The prevailing view at the time was that medical care should be given only to those who survived their first year and who then showed promise of good mental function.

Technical advances in anesthesia, perinatal surgery and in shunts to drain excess fluid from the brain improved the prospects of early intervention. In the late 1950s and early 1960s a group in Sheffield, England, showed that early surgery dramatically increased the survival of a newborn with spina bifida. Enthusiasm for aggressive treatment quickly spread, and most infants with spina bifida were treated. In contrast to the situation with Down syndrome, technology led to the rapid change in treatment of spina bifida.

In 1971 Dr. John Lorber, one of the leaders of the Sheffield group, reviewed his experience with the children he had treated. He concluded that, since half the children given vigorous therapy died anyway and a substantial portion of the survivors were severely impaired, not all such infants should be treated. He suggested selection at birth to reduce the resources committed to both those who would die anyway and those who would survive with substantial impairments. Lorber published a series of articles proposing a list of medical indications for selecting those who should not be treated. In this instance, changes in medical practice led to a change in public morality.

The proposed change from virtually obligatory treatment to selection was also widely, but not universally, adopted. Whereas the shift from no treatment to aggressive treatment caused no ethical debate, the notion of selection challenged the "technological imperative," the immediate move from "can do" to "must do." Selection also raised deep ethical questions terribly reminiscent of the Nazi identification of victims. And it challenged physicians, families, and society to clarify the concept of "quality of life."

By the 1980s a consensus emerged in the United States that required the treatment of all but the most severely afflicted babies with spina bifida. Yet this consensus was in turn challenged by technological developments, the first of which came from improvements in antenatal detection of spina bifida and opened the possibility of aborting affected fetuses. Several courts held that informed consent required that pregnant women be told of the availability of prenatal testing. Although such tests could not predict the degree of physical impairment, the number of live births of spina bifida babies plummeted. Spina bifida, like a number of other handicapping conditions, became a minor ripple in the major debate over abortion.

The second technological change was the introduction of new in utero surgical techniques that apparently cure spina bifida in affected fetuses. As we write, such procedures are experimental, expensive, and not widely available.

This will change with time. Situations will then arise in which women refuse both abortion and effective surgery on the fetus they are carrying. Technology will create yet another moral dilemma.

Currently, a major controversy surrounds the use and limits of technology for treating very small premature newborns. Depending on the size of the infant (birth weight one to three pounds) and the gestational age, the survival rate of these premature infants varies from 10 to 90 percent, and the outcome may vary from normal to profoundly mentally handicapped with severe cerebral palsy. There is no national consensus on the treatment of these babies; criteria for treatment vary from center to center and from physician to physician. Unlike the situation of the child with Down syndrome or spina bifida, however, there is rarely one big decision to make, but rather, as in the Castelli case, a series of small decisions. The outcome of each of these smaller decisions is unpredictable and their effects may be cumulative, thus the phrase "nibbling away in the nursery."

From Karen Quinlan to Nancy Cruzan: Technology Extending Unconscious Existence

It was not long ago that the elderly were cared for at home and typically died of pneumonia or the complications of a stroke or heart attack. Pneumonia was once called "the old man's friend." Antibiotics ended that "friendship." At one time the individual who required respiratory support died. When tank respirators became available, they were not suitable for the elderly or for long-term use. The development of good respirators in the 1960s and 1970s has been a boon to many children and adults with acute respiratory problems. Their use has made it possible to extend lives, some even after the ability to function consciously has been irretrievably lost. Nutrition by tube feeding has further increased our ability to prolong life.

Karen Quinlan's was the first case to draw widespread attention to the capacity of modern medicine to sustain irreversibly comatose patients on a respirator. Respirators are now routine in intensive care units, and feeding through tubes to the stomach is an everyday occurrence in hospitals and nursing homes. Access to air and nutrition would seem to be basic, but there are clearly situations where patients can reject them as "heroic" or physicians judge them futile.

When we look at some of the terms in the current debate over discontinuing treatment of the elderly and comatose—advance directives, living wills, death with dignity, heroic measures, vegetative state—it is plain that the argument is far from closure. How can we consider quality of life without starting down the slippery slope toward killing those whose lives are judged lacking in quality? How can we take the rights of incompetent patients seriously without locking ourselves into rigid programs of aggressively treating all such patients no matter what the circumstances?

Although the courts are only one branch of American government, they have been the one most deeply involved with the controversies in medical ethics. When the legislature becomes involved, as in Medicaid funding of abortion or the 1984 amendments to the Child Abuse Act, the courts have been called on to review the law and its application. When the executive has acted, as in the Baby Doe regulations, the action has been quickly challenged in the courts. The courts, for better and worse, have been the main forum in which Americans have argued the most complex issues of medical ethics.

The fact that an issue is brought to court requires that it be structured in a certain way. Courts are more attuned to issues of individual rights than to public policy or social welfare. They worry less about what makes people happy than about whether people's rights are respected. In decisions concerning the care of Karen Quinlan, Joseph Saikewicz, Claire Conroy, Nancy Cruzan, and Sue Ann Lawrance, courts have wrestled with the issue of who has the right to decide and the limits within which court-appointed guardians may act. (Fuller reference to these cases appears in the suggested readings section at the end of Chapter 18. See especially Albert Jonsen, *The Birth of Bioethics*.) A few opinions have called for the courts themselves to be involved in individual cases; most have called for hospitals or nursing homes to set up procedures for making decisions within boundaries established by the courts.

In preparing their decisions, judges have consulted the writings of philosophers and theologians. As a body of significant decisions developed, they have consulted with each other. In its 1990 Cruzan decision, the Supreme Court provided an exhaustive survey of the legal and ethical literature on decision-making for comatose or extremely handicapped individuals. This decision, and the latest version of the Baby Doe regulations (which we quote in the cases of the Castelli baby and Christie, Chapters 12 and 13) move in the direction of recognizing the validity of decision-making procedures outside the courts. Judges are anxious not to get involved in every difficult medical case that comes along. At the same time, the courts have introduced both substantive and procedural guidelines within which families, physicians, and health care facilities can act.

In the Cruzan decision, for example, the Court recognized that the states could establish substantive and procedural rules. Courts are inclined to see issues in terms of rights and to resolve problems by setting up procedures. That is only natural, since courts are themselves systems of procedures to resolve conflict. But they have also recognized that their particular procedures are not necessarily best for resolving medical and moral issues. The advocacy system, which pits one side against another in hopes that conflict will bring out the truth and result in a fair settlement, does not fit medical situations well. In our cases everyone—family, nurses, physicians, hospitals—is a patient advocate. The problem is that they are often advocating conflicting courses of action. Moreover, bringing a case to a public tribunal involves abandoning much of the privacy to which patients and families are normally entitled. Finally, courts are designed to settle conflicts that can be settled nowhere else, and most courts believe that the issues of medical ethics can better be settled by the patients, families, nurses, physicians, and hospitals most directly involved.

In recent years, however, some critics have claimed that medical ethics has degenerated into a compendium of law cases. The attempt to work out a system of rules that would lead to right decisions has led to a single rule for every situation—let the patient decide. Autonomy has become the one-size-fits-all solution. Yet the autonomous individual—self-controlled, in charge, and isolated from social influences—is largely the creation of philosophical imagination. Furthermore, decisions in medicine are not like those of an appellate court that has the leisure to look back over the way in which a completed case was handled. Medical decision-making is prospective, looking toward a future that is necessarily uncertain and risky.

While agreeing in part with this criticism, we take a more positive message from court involvement in medical ethics. Our discussion of the courts and how they have dealt with the issues provides an important clue to constructive moral thinking. Good moral thinking depends on something akin to procedure. Since, as several of our cases illustrate, people must often live with bad outcomes, how decisions are made is the critical ingredient of their goodness. We can only face such outcomes if we are satisfied with the process that we used for the decisions that contributed to the outcomes.

Making Good Decisions

Good decisions are marked by openness to all the medical information that is available, to the patient and to all who are involved with the patient's care, whether as relatives or as professionals, and to the cultures, subcultures, and society of which the patient is a member. Some use *openness* as a code word for moral relativism, and in turn use relativism to escape moral evaluation. We think of openness as just the opposite: it is a practical instrument of moral evaluation and self-criticism.

The historical events we have discussed show how people can close themselves off from a morally significant aspect of a medical and human situation. The Nazis ignored the humanity of their victims, and some instances of allowing newborns with Down syndrome to die came frighteningly close to that.

Patients, family members, physicians, and nurses sometimes try to exclude legitimately involved persons from decisions.

Good, open decisions rely on good facts or at least on the best knowledge currently available. Physicians are not omniscient, but they are responsible for obtaining the latest and most accurate medical information. Good decisions are also open both to the views of others involved in the situation and to outside opinion. In this way the decision makers are assured of multiple points of view and become aware of their own bias. This also means that varied ethical theories will enter into the decision-making process.

We differ from rule-based moral theorists, either utilitarians or deontologists, in thinking that good decision-making processes can come to different conclusions in essentially identical cases. This does not mean, however, that any answer will do or even that a widely based social consensus is necessarily correct. What was once widely accepted treatment of the mentally handicapped is now recognized as morally deficient.

Tolerance is the public or political dimension of the open decision-making we advocate. Differences in viewpoint and value are inherent in the complex moral and human situations confronting medical ethics. Tolerance involves being open to those differences. As our historical examples show, excluding values or legitimately interested parties from consideration leads to the narrowness of view that characterizes bad actions.

Unfortunately, tolerance too often is identified with moral relativism or lack of clarity in ethical theory. We see tolerance as a middle ground between dogmatism on the one hand and moral relativism on the other. Dogmatism can take many forms, only some of which are readily recognizable. Lucille Adams (in the case of Christie) represents one form of dogmatism insofar as she might demand aggressive treatment of every newborn no matter how poor the prognosis or painful and crippling the treatment. Dr. Bernstein (in the case of the Castelli baby) exhibits a similar dogmatism when he advocates using all available medical technology. But equally dogmatic are those who would give parents complete discretion in making decisions for their children. Even an exclusive focus on informed consent and patient autonomy can become a form of dogmatism. We differ with those who hold that there is a uniquely correct person to make moral decisions. These apparently different attitudes share a common failure in fastening on a single aspect of a complex moral situation and proceeding to make it into *the* moral absolute—the single key answer to all moral questions.

The whole point of tolerance is setting limits. Failure to treat a child with a mildly handicapping condition is intolerable: it ignores the child's potential for a fulfilling life. While we are more inclined to tolerate aggressive treatment than unjustifiable nontreatment, there is no sufficient reason to tolerate futile and painful treatment of surely fatal diseases, even when patients or relatives demand that "something be done."

Although physicians may tolerate wide divergences in the decisions of their patients, they have an obligation to assure that both the patients and they themselves understand the risks, benefits, and likely consequences of a proposed course of action. Physicians also must decide whether a patient's decisions are within that physician's own limits of tolerance. If a physician cannot accept a patient's decision, then he or she should withdraw from the case and refer the patient to another physician.

While tolerance is a relatively passive virtue, the active virtue of medicine is beneficence. Medicine is a helping profession, striving to produce benefits for patients. Physicians and nurses try to meet the needs of others, but an excess of beneficence may overwhelm patients and lead to paternalism. Although the beneficent actions of medical professionals have generally served both patients and society well, the technological power of modern medicine easily can convert beneficence to arrogance. With growing confidence in their ability to help patients, physicians sometimes help them to live or die in ways those individuals disapprove.

Both the general public and the philosophical community have complained of the arrogance of medicine. Some want physicians to restrict themselves to purely technical matters and refrain from bringing their human perspective to the patient's decision-making. We think this attitude pushes the pendulum too far. Decisions should be made both by patients, with the advice and consent of their caregivers, and by physicians, with the consent of their well-informed patients. Physicians possess enormous power to shape patients' decisions both by what they tell them and by what they do not say. Their tone of voice, their emphasis on the positive or negative, their body language, and all that is involved in human communication structure the information patients receive. At the same time, patients can withdraw from a physician's care. More subtly, patients can refuse to comply with prescribed treatment, distort their report of symptoms, or in other ways frustrate their physicians' efforts on their behalf. None of this leads to good medicine.

Good decisions result from an interactive, even symbiotic, relationship between physician and patient. The relationship also includes family members, friends, nurses, and other members of the health care team. All participants in the process must work within the limits of their own tolerance. This is true both for decisions to limit and for decisions to start treatment. Good processes of decision-making require that all parties tolerate the diversity of others' viewpoints and work toward defining and achieving a consensus about what is best for the patient.

The classical discussion of medical ethics focused on the Hippocratic tradition and emphasized acting for the benefit of the patient. Abuses of beneficence such as the paternalism of well-intentioned but authoritarian physicians helped bring autonomy and informed consent to the fore as a counterbalance. The principle of autonomy was readily accepted because it connects so closely with the traditions of liberty that inform political discussion in the United States.

In rushing to insure individual liberty and autonomy, however, our culture is in some danger of moving to an opposite extreme. We too often, it seems, ignore the fact that the principal barrier to a patient's liberty is debilitating disease. When it restores health, medicine restores freedom as well. Over-emphasizing the right of patients to refuse medical care can obscure the benefits of effective medicine. At this time we are less afraid of a little paternalism than we are of the social isolation and neglect of good health care that can follow from too much emphasis on autonomy.

We are concerned that a balance be restored. Given the difficulties of conveying meaningful medical information to patients and the inevitable limits that disease imposes on freedom and autonomy, informed consent is not, by itself, adequate to insure morally good decisions. The beneficent tradition of medicine needs to be recognized as the engine that drives researchers and caregivers to help those who depend on them. It is an irreplaceable element of good morals and good medicine.

Most of all, however, we are heartened by the success of medical ethics over the past 25 years in opening these issues to public discussion and debate. Philosophers, physicians, patients, nurses, and many others have weighed in with their concerns and points of view. Legislatures, state governors, U.S. presidents, and especially the courts have played a prominent role. Physicians, philosophers, and theologians have participated in the discussions on local ethics committees and review boards. All is not perfect, nor will it ever be. But there is, in the U.S. now, a widespread tolerance for people's different views of life and its meaning, and also some consensus about the limits of that tolerance, of things we will not permit. The specifics will change, but it is the process of that change that will be morally significant.